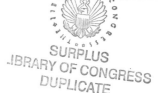
# Handbook of
# Career Development
# in Academic Psychiatry
# and Behavioral Sciences

# Handbook of Career Development in Academic Psychiatry and Behavioral Sciences

Edited by

Laura Weiss Roberts, M.D., M.A.
Donald M. Hilty, M.D.

Sponsored by the

*Association for Academic Psychiatry*

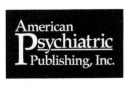

Washington, DC
London, England

Copyright © 2006 American Psychiatric Publishing, Inc.
ALL RIGHTS RESERVED

Typeset in Adobe's HelveticaNeue and Palatino.

Manufactured in the United States of America on acid-free paper.
08  07  06  05  04      5  4  3  2  1
First Edition

American Psychiatric Publishing, Inc.
1000 Wilson Boulevard
Arlington, VA 22209-3901
www.appi.org

**Library of Congress Cataloging-in-Publication Data**

Handbook of career development in academic psychiatry and behavioral
sciences / [edited by] Laura Weiss Roberts, Donald M. Hilty.-- 1st ed.
    p. ; cm. -- (Concise guides series)
  Includes bibliographical references and index.
  ISBN 1-58562-208-7 (pbk. : alk. paper)
  1. Psychiatry--Study and teaching--Vocational guidance. 2. Psychology--Study
and teaching--Vocational guidance. 3. Psychiatry--Research--Vocational guidance. 4. Psychology--Research--Vocational guidance. 5. Career development.
  [DNLM: 1. Psychiatry--Handbooks. 2. Behavioral Sciences--Handbooks. WM
34 H2353 2005] I. Roberts, Laura Weiss, 1960- II. Hilty, Donald M., 1964-.
  RC459.5.U6.H35 2005
  616.89'0071--dc22

2005014184

**British Library Cataloguing in Publication Data**
A CIP record is available from the British Library.

# Contents

## PART I

### Getting Started...

# PART II

## Getting There...

# PART III

## Once You're There...

# PART IV

## Becoming an Educator...

# PART V

## Developing Your Academic Skills...

# PART VI

## Continuing to Grow
## Professionally...

# Contributors

**Jerald Belitz, Ph.D.**
Associate Professor and Chief Psychologist and Clinical Director of Children's Psychiatric Center/Outpatient Services, Department of Psychiatry, University of New Mexico School of Medicine, Albuquerque, New Mexico

**Jonathan F. Borus, M.D.**
Chair, Department of Psychiatry, Brigham and Women's/Faulkner Hospitals; Stanley Cobb Professor of Psychiatry, Harvard Medical School, Boston, Massachusetts

**James A. Clardy, M.D.**
Professor of Psychiatry, Associate Dean for Graduate Medical Education, College of Medicine, University of Arkansas for Medical Sciences, Little Rock, Arkansas

**Blythe A. Corbett, Ph.D.**
Assistant Clinical Professor, Department of Psychiatry and Behavioral Sciences, University of California–Davis, Sacramento, California

**John H. Coverdale, M.D., M.Ed., FRANZCP**
Associate Professor, Menninger Department of Psychiatry, Baylor College of Medicine, Houston, Texas

**Laura B. Dunn, M.D.**
Assistant Professor of Psychiatry, Department of Psychiatry, University of California–San Diego, San Diego, California

**Kristin Edenharder, B.A.**
Assistant Editor, Department of Psychiatry and Behavioral Medicine, Medical College of Wisconsin, Milwaukee, Wisconsin

**Cynthia M.A. Geppert, M.D., Ph.D.**
Assistant Professor, Department of Psychiatry, University of New Mexico School of Medicine; Chief, Consultation-Liaison Psychiatry and Ethics, New Mexico Veterans Affairs Health Care System, Albuquerque, New Mexico

**Richard H. Gibson, M.D.**
Assistant Professor, Department of Psychiatry and Behavioral Medicine; Division Manager, Milwaukee VA Medical Center, Medical College of Wisconsin, Milwaukee, Wisconsin

**Brad K. Grunert, Ph.D.**
Associate Professor, Plastic Surgery, Froedtert West Clinics, Milwaukee, Wisconsin

**Deborah J. Hales, M.D.**
Director, Division of Education, American Psychiatric Association, Arlington, Virginia

**Robert E. Hales, M.D., M.B.A.**
Professor and Chair, Department of Psychiatry and Behavioral Sciences, University of California–Davis, Sacramento, California

**Thomas Heinrich, M.D.**
Assistant Professor, Department of Psychiatry and Behavioral Medicine, Medical College of Wisconsin, Milwaukee, Wisconsin

**Donald M. Hilty, M.D.**
Associate Professor of Clinical Psychiatry, Department of Psychiatry and Behavioral Sciences, University of California–Davis, Sacramento, California

**Joseph B. Layde, M.D., J.D.**
Associate Professor, Department of Psychiatry and Behavioral Medicine, Medical College of Wisconsin, Milwaukee, Wisconsin

**Martin H. Leamon, M.D.**
Associate Professor of Clinical Psychiatry, Department of Psychiatry and Behavioral Sciences, University of California–Davis, Sacramento, California

**Jon Lehrmann, M.D.**
Assistant Professor, Department of Psychiatry and Behavioral Medicine, Medical College of Wisconsin; Program Manager, Milwaukee Veterans Affairs Medical Center, Milwaukee, Wisconsin

**Russell F. Lim, M.D.**
Associate Clinical Professor, Director of Diversity Education and Training, Department of Psychiatry and Behavioral Sciences, University of California–Davis, Sacramento, California

**Alan Louie, M.D.**
Director, Psychiatry Residency Training Program, San Mateo County Mental Health Services; Clinical Professor, University of California Medical Center, San Francisco, California

**Teresita McCarty, M.D.**
Director of Assessment, University of New Mexico School of Medicine, Department of Psychiatry, Albuquerque, New Mexico

**Dan-Vy Mui, M.D.**
Assistant Professor and Director of Consult Liaison, University of Arkansas for Medical Sciences, Department of Psychiatry, Little Rock, Arkansas

**Andrew Norton, M.D.**
Associate Professor of Medicine, General Internal Medicine, Medical College of Wisconsin, Milwaukee, Wisconsin

**Carlos N. Pato, M.D.**
Associate Chief of Staff, Research and Development, Veterans Affairs Medical Center, Washington, D.C.; Distinguished Professor of Psychiatry, Georgetown University Hospital and School of Medicine, Washington, D.C.; Professor of Psychiatry, State University of New York-Upstate Medical University, Syracuse, New York

**Michele T. Pato, M.D.**
Associate Chief of Staff, Department of Education, Veterans Affairs Medical Center, Washington, D.C.; Director of Education-Psychiatry, Georgetown University Hospital and School of Medicine, Washington, D.C.; Professor of Psychiatry, State University of New York-Upstate Medical University, Center for NeuroPsychiatric Genetics, Syracuse, New York

**David Peterson, M.B.A., FACMPE**
Department Administrator, Department of Psychiatry and Behavioral Medicine, Medical College of Wisconsin, Milwaukee, Wisconsin

**Annelle B. Primm, M.D., M.P.H.**
Director, Minority and National Affairs, American Psychiatric Association, Arlington, Virginia

**Laura Weiss Roberts, M.D., M.A.**
Professor and Chair, Department of Psychiatry and Behavioral Medicine, Medical College of Wisconsin, Milwaukee, Wisconsin

**Stephen Scheiber, M.D.**
Executive Vice President, American Board of Psychiatry and Neurology, Deerfield, Illinois

**Deborah Simpson, Ph.D.**
Associate Dean for Educational Support and Evaluation, Professor, Family and Community Medicine, and Director, Office of Educational Services, Medical College of Wisconsin, Milwaukee, Wisconsin

**Ryan Spellecy, Ph.D.**
Assistant Professor of Bioethics, Center for the Study of Bioethics, and Assistant Professor, Department of Psychiatry and Behavioral Medicine, Medical College of Wisconsin, Milwaukee, Wisconsin

**Malathi Srinivasan, M.D.**
Assistant Professor of Medicine and Robert Wood Johnson Foundation Faculty Scholar, Department of General Medicine, University of California–Davis, Sacramento, California

**Hendry Ton, M.D.**
Assistant Clinical Professor, Department of Psychiatry and Behavioral Sciences, University of California–Davis, Sacramento, California

**Teddy D. Warner, Ph.D.**
Research Associate Professor, Department of Family and Community Medicine, University of New Mexico School of Medicine, Albuquerque, New Mexico

**Michael S. Wilkes, M.D.**
Associate Dean of Medical Education, University of California–Davis, School of Medicine, Sacramento, California

## Linda L.M. Worley, M.D.

Associate Professor, Departments of Psychiatry and Obstetrics and Gynecology, University of Arkansas for Medical Sciences, Little Rock, Arkansas

## Joel Yager, M.D.

Professor, Department of Psychiatry, University of New Mexico School of Medicine, Albuquerque, New Mexico

# Preface

There are about a million things we wish someone had taught us, told us, or at least hinted at when we started our academic careers. Traditional medical training did not prepare us for writing letters of recommendation, creating or understanding budgets, giving difficult feedback, interviewing for jobs, teaching, negotiating with department chairs, writing test questions, networking, or, frankly, most of the things that—as it turns out—academic faculty members do all the time. This book is filled with a lot of those things. We hope you will find it to be a valuable tool. Most important, we hope it will save you valuable time so that you may be effective, experience joy, and find success in your professional life.

Laura Weiss Roberts, M.D., M.A.
Donald M. Hilty, M.D.

# Acknowledgments

The editors express their heartfelt appreciation to the editorial assistant for this work, Ms. Kristin Edenharder. We deeply thank the authors whose wonderful contributions populate this book, and Dr. Robert E. Hales and Mr. John McDuffie of American Psychiatric Publishing, Inc., for their enthusiasm for this unique project.

Dr. Roberts wishes to express her thanks and love to her mother (and hero), Anne Weisskopf, her husband, Brian, and her children, Tommy, Willa, Helen, and Madeline, all of whom are very nice to put up with her. She further thanks her friend and co-editor, Dr. Donald Hilty, whose collegiality, professionalism, and effort made this endeavor much more fun than work.

Dr. Hilty wishes to express his thanks to his parents, siblings, and daughter, Sarah. He greatly appreciates the collaboration of colleagues at University of California–Davis, and those in the Association for Academic Psychiatry, Association of American Directors of Psychiatry Residency Training, and American Directors of Medical Student Education in Psychiatry. Finally, he thanks Dr. Laura Roberts for her inspiring leadership, organization, and collaborative spirit.

The editors wish to acknowledge the wonderful assistance of Mr. Mark Talatzko and Ms. Karen Hamilton in the preparation of this manuscript.

# PART I

# Getting Started…

# CHAPTER 1

# Approaching Your Academic Career

Laura Weiss Roberts, M.D., M.A.

Donald M. Hilty, M.D.

Success…is a result, not a goal.

*Gustave Flaubert*

Very few of us approach our academic careers methodically and with great foresight, and even the most accomplished leaders in academic medicine are often surprised at where their professional efforts, and serendipity, have taken them. Our impression is that the most fulfilling, robust academic careers in our field are those that have been shaped by certain attributes of the faculty member as well as the context for the individual's professional development. These attributes are described in this chapter, as are strategies for the faculty member who aspires to a positive academic career path.

## ATTRIBUTES OF THE FACULTY MEMBER

There are a few key qualities that we have observed in colleagues whose careers can be characterized as having greatly contributed to our profession and as having earned the genuine respect of their peers.

> The whole secret of a successful life is to find out what it is one's destiny to do, and then do it.
>
> *Henry Ford*

The first of these qualities is the most important: a *sense of purpose* or a professional calling. It may be teaching. It may be healing. It may be finding answers to questions that matter. It may be creating, nurturing, or communicating. It may be serving in a manner that allows others to become fulfilled and to make their own contribution. Seeing the relationship between the everyday work activities of a faculty member and their broader meaning is vital to staying motivated in academia. In this way, the faculty member's professional effort isn't reduced to just another lecture to give, on call night to survive, IRB proposal to submit, experiment to run, set of data to analyze, performance evaluation to complete, or QA report to do.

This concept of meaningfulness is linked with an understanding of why academic departments of psychiatry and behavioral sciences have a unique role in our society. Though a well-run department and successful faculty often draw from the principles of business, ours is not just another business. Our departments are entrusted with preparing the next generation of physicians and scientists, with generating new knowledge of importance to human experience, and with serving people and communities to improve health. These responsibilities and aims differ from those of other organizations in our society.

An academic faculty member is part of this unique endeavor; the faculty member as teacher, clinician, scientist, administrator, mentor, and advocate thus becomes the willing "means" through which things that matter may be accomplished. Explicit attention to this sense of purpose on the part of faculty, both as individuals and as members of our academic institutions, has done much to inspire many very remarkable careers in our field.

> It took me twenty years to become an overnight success.
>
> *Eddie Cantor*

> At no time am I a quick thinker or writer: whatever I have done...has solely been by long pondering, patience, and industry.
>
> *Charles Darwin*

A second quality is willingness to engage in *hard work*. Serving as an academic faculty member involves considerable responsibility to patients, learners, colleagues, supervisors, organizations, and communities. Often early career faculty members are in front-line positions that involve responding to many pressing needs. It is not unusual for multidisciplinary professionals to work as hard in their first few years on faculty as they did during their training years, if not harder. For these reasons, being an early career faculty member is very effortful, entailing exertion that is disciplined, sustained, and thoughtfully directed.

It is also important that, whenever possible, these intense efforts give rise to tangible work products. The advantage of this is certainly clear with respect to generating manuscripts for peer review, grant applications, and policy documents. But it is also true that producing more modest "local" documents has its advantages. For instance, a well-conceived, well-written summary report with practical recommendations will help ensure that a positive committee process has a valuable and enduring impact. Such documents also concretely demonstrate one's commitment to working toward shared goals, doing much to establish one's "good citizenship" with colleagues. Under many circumstances, these work products may be included in one's annual review documents, teaching portfolio, or curriculum vitae.

> It's not work, if you love what you're doing.
>
> *Steve Sears*

> In order to create there must be a dynamic force, and what force is more potent than love?
>
> *Igor Stravinsky*

> Knowing a lot…is a springboard to creativity.
>
> *Charlie Rose*

A third quality of successful faculty is *creativity*, an attribute that is seldom recognized for its importance in clinical service, education, and administration. Creativity gives rise to valuable activities and resources, acting as a platform for translating knowledge into true expertise. The creative process itself provides a feeling of joy and even artistry that can give much emotional sustenance to the faculty member who might otherwise feel depleted by the demands of professional life. Through creativity, work is transformed from mere industry to tasks that represent something one loves and finds fulfillment in.

*Being organized* is essential in order to be an effective, accomplished faculty member. For some people, this seems very natural—making lists of things to do and then delightedly and relentlessly ticking off each item is just great fun. For others, creating a system for remembering things, finishing things, and following up on things is much more of a challenge. The key is to recognize that being well organized creates time and freedom; inventing ways of being more effective aids in keeping up with one's obligations and feeling less stressed.

> The secret of success is constancy of purpose.
>
> *Benjamin Disraeli*

> Success is relative: it is what we can make of the mess we have made of things.
>
> *T.S. Eliot*

The next quality is a combination of *tenacity* and *resilience*. Early in an academic career, a faculty member is tested, stretched, pushed, and pulled in his or her efforts to meet the demands of the position. Assuming this new role means developing new skills, encountering new challenges and novel situations, and taking measured but definite risks. Attaining some measure of mastery will involve staying with things, even if they are difficult and do not come easily or quickly. The gains are considerable: when we try a variety of experiences early on, it helps us define interests, develop skills, and meet others with shared interests.

A great example of the importance of tenacity and resilience is the process of getting a paper published or a grant funded. Almost no one has a manuscript accepted without first being rejected. It is important to view the initial submission step as an opportunity to get feedback and to strengthen one's scholarly work. Similarly, almost no one gets a grant funded without first having written an unsuccessful application. The opportunity to learn from—and improve one's work through—the careful critiques provided in a grant review process is much more important than the initial outcome of a single proposal.

> The only way to have a friend is to be one.
>
> *Ralph Waldo Emerson*

> Friendships multiply joys and divide griefs.
>
> *Thomas Fuller*

The ability to build a *reservoir of good will* in one's professional life is another important attribute of a successful faculty member. In our experience, good will is fostered by collegiality, promise-keeping, authenticity,
and repeated acts of generosity. Sacrificing one's best interests for the
sake of others is not necessary but, on the other hand, an exclusive
"what's in it for me?" attitude will rapidly diminish a career with great
potential. Good will creates a more supportive and forgiving environment for professional development and collaboration, even in the face
of the adversity, competition, or divisive pressures that may be encountered over the long span of an academic career.

> I've always been in the right place at the right
> time. Of course, I steered myself there.
>
> *Bob Hope*

> If at first you don't succeed, try, try again.
> Then quit. No use being a damn fool about it.
>
> *W.C. Fields*

> Everyone must row with the oars he has.
>
> *Anonymous*

There is no single word to characterize the final quality that we wish to
highlight of an accomplished academic faculty member; it is the blend-
ing of *insight, intuition,* and *openness to opportunity.* The most successful
faculty members are not the most brilliant ones; rather, they are the ones
who understand their strengths and know how to work with and overcome their weaknesses, who know how to find roles where they can be
effective and valued, and who are willing to take the right kinds of risks
and know when to pull back from the wrong kinds of commitments.
They are individuals who discern possibilities that others may be less
sensitive to, and who trust their ability to read complex situations.
These factors, in turn, lead others to have confidence in them, thus creating new opportunities. A chance meeting at a national conference may
lead to a series of manuscripts, workshops, and other collaborations. An
unexpected assignment to a committee may introduce a faculty member
to a new set of issues, a new body of literature, or a new set of colleagues. Interviewing for a position in another city may lead to a new
way of thinking about your current post. These are all potential professional developmental opportunities—occasions for learning about one's
self and one's situation. Some people develop the gift for seeing the

possibilities in circumstances earlier than others, but we believe that this is a quality that can be cultivated, for instance, through self-reflection, observation of the career paths of colleagues, and discussion with one's mentors.

## THE CONTEXT FOR PROFESSIONAL DEVELOPMENT

> It is the supreme art of the teacher to awaken joy in creative expression and knowledge.
>
> *Albert Einstein*

> A teacher's major contribution may pop out anonymously in the life of some ex-student's grandchild.
>
> *Wendell Berry*

Wonderful careers happen all over; there is no perfect or even necessary context for professional development. This observation is supported by many examples of accomplished academicians whose careers have been "incubated" in any number of very different professional situations.

Nevertheless, there are important features that characterize advantageous environments for professional development (see Chapter 29). The first is having mentors or "coaches" present in the immediate environment. An effective mentoring relationship is critical in providing advice on how and when to do what in one's academic career. For instance, each institution possesses its own set of written rules and requirements for promotion and tenure and its own unspoken institutional culture. A good mentor (see Chapter 26) will help you understand both the formal and the informal ways that academia works and will help you stay focused on activities that will benefit your career. In addition, association with a good mentor will enhance your reputation. Mentorship has been long recognized as vital to a mentee's achieving higher levels of career satisfaction, promotion, publications, confidence in his or her capabilities, research productivity, and financial success. Just as important, a mentor will help you to get through tough times in career development, whether personal or professional in nature.

> I educate, not by lessons, but by going about my business.
>
> *Socrates*

A good boss is important, too. Faculty need to balance their individual goals with those of the department and the school of medicine in order to be successful. Often, shifts in commitments and goals occur as the faculty member progresses through his or her career. Division leaders and department chairs who understand the importance of balancing the organizational and professional development needs of their faculty are wonderful resources. A word of encouragement, the ability to attend a conference, the "green light" to pursue an idea or project, accurate feedback to help improve performance—these are all important moments in the career of a faculty member.

> The freedom to make mistakes provides the best environment for creativity.
>
> *Anonymous*

An advantageous academic environment will provide diverse opportunities for learning. This means there will be sufficient complexity in the environment to allow for new challenges, sufficient autonomy to explore one's interests and abilities, and sufficient resources (interpersonal, material) to provide some measure of protection (e.g., time, supportive supervision) for professional growth and development. For instance, faculty members engage in many activities at a university or in other academic settings that can be categorized into five general areas: clinical, research, teaching, administrative, and community service. Some of these may feel like a good fit for early career faculty, while others may be quite unfamiliar. Also, the faculty member may not be completely sure what he or she wants to do. In that case, early career faculty try a mix of activities to clarify interests—and, in the process, help the department meet its needs as well as its service obligations to the community.

This approach works well as long as there is an understanding that priorities may change over time for both the faculty member and the department. Often, too, things change (e.g., a decrease in contracts or grants, the departures of key collaborators, the promotion of a division head or department chair). As in the investment world, where it is important to have a diversified portfolio, it is helpful to have a marketable area (or two) of expertise that is adaptable to various changes. Another key to versatility is building relationships with many individuals—and not to the exclusion of anyone. A good environment for professional development will have enough complexity that opportunities such as these are truly possible.

One of the things that we value most about our field is that there are many ways to thrive and to contribute—there are many paths. The individual's own attributes and his or her fit with the resources and possibilities in the context, taken together, create the platform for academic faculty development.

## SMART STRATEGIES

- Find opportunities where you can be yourself and join others doing the things you enjoy.
- Try new experiences—within reason—to define your interests and meet others.
- Find support from other faculty, friends, and mentors.
- Find the tools you need to be organized and time-efficient.
- Take a good look at your colleagues and mentors: What can you learn from their career choices? What can you learn from their successes and failures?
- Think hard about the strengths and potential obstacles for growth in your present environment.
- Consider your career in 2- to 5-year increments, and think about specific accomplishments that you may wish to pursue during each period.

## QUESTIONS TO DISCUSS WITH A MENTOR OR COLLEAGUE

1. What are the predictable choice-points in an academic career path?
2. What are my greatest strengths, and what in my current environment fosters my professional development?
3. What are my greatest weaknesses, and what in my current environment fails to foster my professional development?
4. What professionals can I talk to about the lessons they have learned over the course of their careers?
5. What are the "unwritten rules" in our department and our institution?

## ADDITIONAL RESOURCES

Heim P, Golant SK: Hardball for Women: Winning at the Game of Business. New York, Plume, 1993

# Strategies for Academically Oriented Residents in Psychiatry

Laura B. Dunn, M.D.

This chapter focuses on overall and specific strategies for residents and fellows who have an interest in pursuing academic careers in psychiatry. Important considerations addressed in this chapter include choosing a residency, fellowship, or department; specific strategies for each phase of residency; choosing a mentor; assessing your interests and temperament and how these fit with types of career paths in academic psychiatry (i.e., to help determine how best to combine clinical, research, teaching, and administrative ambitions and responsibilities); and developing an informed, yet flexible, perspective as you pursue your career development.

## CHOOSING A RESIDENCY, FELLOWSHIP, OR DEPARTMENT

As a key decision point in an early career, the choice of residency or fellowship program deserves careful consideration. When selecting a residency, fellowship, or department, consider your personal needs and preferences, and examine programs carefully with these in mind (see Chapter 6). Specific considerations will differ for an intern or resident compared to those of a junior faculty member, yet the major themes are the same. For instance, it may be clear at an early stage of training that you prefer a more research-oriented program or a program that is more clinically focused.

As a first step, be sure to investigate a broad range of programs. Then, when interviewing at each institution, meet with as many individuals as possible and try to arrange to meet with people whose work particularly interests you. This kind of information is often available online, and doing your homework prior to interviews—by having a general idea of faculty members' focus—is well received and shows initiative.

For incoming residents or fellows considering a career in academic psychiatry, there are several key features to look for in a program. A program should offer opportunities to work with established mentors (who have enough time to work with you; more on that later); to gain teaching, writing, research, and administrative experience; and to pursue specialized fellowships in your area of interest. If, like most of us starting out, you are unsure of which specific areas within academic psychiatry will be your future home, it is best to try to find a program with a broad range of opportunities, with mentors who can help you hone a variety of skills.

Consider whether you want a more structured program, where the curriculum is essentially preset for residents for their entire four years, or one where the residents have considerable leeway to shape their own schedules, particularly in the latter years. Ask about special research tracks for residents and what they actually mean in practice: is the time "protected," and how is this accomplished? For residents particularly interested in developing expertise in teaching, ask about opportunities to teach medical students (in addition to those students who rotate on the clinical services). Fellowships may offer time for research or teaching endeavors, but it is important to find out how well this time is protected in practice, what kinds of projects fellows have completed, and whether there is any administrative or technical support available (e.g., retrieving articles from the library). It is important to ask about these matters tactfully, however. You must present yourself as willing and eager to put in the upfront investment of time and energy required to start a career in academic psychiatry.

Looking at the track records of graduates will also help you determine which programs are most successful at launching academic psychiatrists. This information may or may not be easy to access, but asking faculty about this can be useful. Also, if you have an interest in research, ask to meet with residents who are currently doing research. Ask plenty of questions, while being courteous and appreciative of the time people have spent with you.

Consider the issue of mentorship during your visit, and ask those you meet (when appropriate) about the atmosphere and track record of the department with regard to mentorship (see Chapter 26 in this volume).

In addition to the issues described above, a primary issue to consider is to what degree a department's values mesh with your own. That is, in addition to its reputation, resources, caliber of faculty and residents, and number of grant dollars, there are less tangible aspects meriting consideration. These include such issues as the overall atmosphere, collegiality, supportiveness, and flexibility of a department. This is not to imply that it is easy to gauge these qualities during a brief visit, but rather that it is important to think about these domains when getting a sense of how you would fit into a department. Consider also the general academic environment (is it a public or a private institution, and how does this variable affect the faculty?); history of promotion of junior faculty; and history of funding and other forms of start-up support for junior faculty (see Chapter 10).

Depending on how precisely you know your current and future career interests, you can consider a variety of strategies for assessing programs and departments and finding one that best matches your needs and preferences. For example, if you have a strong interest in combining teaching with a career in clinical psychiatry, finding a program with a strong tradition of valuing this career path will be important. Likewise for aspiring researchers: finding a psychiatry faculty member in your current institution who can help you assess departments is a recommended starting point and can be invaluable. So, make appointments to talk to people, thank them for their time, and do your homework! These initial investments will be time well spent.

## MENTORSHIP

The qualities of a good mentor have been described in some detail (Cohen 1999), but obviously your own individual needs will determine who will be the best match. It is very useful to have several mentors who have complementary skills: one may be more supportive or accepting or may be able to provide more general career guidance; others are more structured in their approach, setting deadlines and helping you prioritize projects or goals. Your primary mentor should be the person with whom you are conducting research, writing papers, or working on other specific, content-related projects. Your other mentors' specific research or clinical and teaching interests do not need to match your own, but these individuals too must be willing and able to help you develop your priorities and career plan.

First and foremost, however, you must be aware of and prepared to meet the requirements of being a good mentee. The mentor must be able to gauge your progress in meeting identifiable goals. Setting up a semi-annual or annual contract can be very useful. The contract can specify detailed goals and timelines in relation to projects (e.g., papers, studies, teaching activities); it can also establish priorities for skills to work on during different time periods. Again, your taking the initiative to suggest, develop, and implement such a plan may be very much appreciated by your mentors (see Chapter 26 for more on mentorship).

## STRATEGIES DURING RESIDENCY

### PGY1 and 2

This time period should be spent exploring opportunities in your department, and searching for mentors. Given the constraints on your time during the first 2 years, don't worry too much about getting started on an actual research project. Instead, think of this time as a chance to shop around, explore your options, and gather information about who will be the best mentors for you. Most faculty members are happy to have genuinely interested and hard-working residents get involved in their research. Many faculty have projects they'd like to do and papers they'd like to write but are constrained themselves by time and energy.

Having chosen your mentor or mentors, this is the time to start immersing yourself in the literature of your chosen topic area, reading broadly for general background and exploring specific interests in more detail. Do not focus in too narrowly at this point. You may need to be judicious as well about what projects you agree to; this is why it is useful to have more than one mentor. Writing reviews and chapters is generally useful at this point because it forces you to amass all of the relevant literature on a specific topic, synthesize ideas, and write.

These 2 years are also crucial for the development of teaching and evaluation skills. Try to learn to be organized about working with medical students: hold weekly meetings with your students, and practice giving mini-lectures to them on topics of interest. You should also practice giving feedback, an important but often avoided task. Learn about the qualities of good teachers, particularly in the medical context, and start practicing these skills and habits. An excellent resource for developing your teaching skills is the Residents' Teaching Skills Web site (http://www.ucimc.netouch.com), which was developed by the University of California, Irvine, in collaboration with the Graduate Medical Education (GME) Section of the Association of American Medical Colleges (AAMC). The Web site also includes an extensive bibliography (http://www.ucimc.netouch.com/bibliography.shtml).

## PGY3 and 4

This is the critical period for developing mentoring relationships. Solidifying mentoring relationships within your own institution (and formalizing these relationships) is vital, but it is also important to begin networking outside of your institution, whether or not you think you will be staying on there in some capacity after residency. This is because recognition by peers and senior faculty outside your institution is a key component of academic success and is one way in which your career development will be measured by your evaluators.

There should be time in these years to write at least one review paper, and ideally one or more data-based papers, using either your own or someone else's data (under his or her supervision). This will most likely require substantial time outside of regular working hours. (Consider that if you are not prepared to put in this time now, then academic psychiatry may not be for you.) Other writing opportunities to seek include helping more senior people write chapters or invited papers and gaining some practice reviewing manuscripts. Attending national meetings and applying for honors, awards, and special fellowships through national organizations is also important at this time.

During your fourth year, you should ideally try to carve out some dedicated time (the amount available and the timing will of course depend on the individual department) for your scholarly endeavors. If you are striving to become a "clinician-educator," you can offer to teach medical students and interns in formal settings; this will provide invaluable experience in mastering subject areas and learning to communicate knowledge and skills to learners. Also strive to learn more about how to evaluate learners and how to give and seek feedback. Also important is to begin developing your writing habits; this means making time to write and consciously working on writing skills.

Gaining experience at writing research plans and submitting proposals to your human subjects review program (institutional review board) is very important if you have a research focus; make sure to be involved at *every* level of your research if you are starting a new study or taking on part of someone else's program of study. Learning to navigate the often complex system of institutional review, protocol safeguards, and grant submission machinery is extremely important because it is the bread and butter of every researcher.

Table 2–1 provides a synthesis of the discussion above, outlining major goals and areas of focus throughout the residency period. Table 2–2 summarizes academic orientations and the kinds of skills that you can begin to hone during residency in preparation for an academic career.

## GENERAL STRATEGIES

### Joining Organizations

Joining the American Psychiatric Association (APA), and other smaller organizations, is a smart and, in many ways, critical step toward success in a career in academic psychiatry (see Chapter 27). Large organizations such as APA provide many diverse opportunities for involvement in various professionally important activities. However, some of the best professional networking opportunities emerge from involvement in smaller organizations. These organizations range from those focused on education (e.g., the Association for Academic Psychiatry, the American College of Psychiatry, and the American Association of Directors of Psychiatric Residency Training [AADPRT]) to those committed to subspecialty psychiatric research, education, and practice issues (e.g., the American Association for Geriatric Psychiatry, the American Academy of Child and Adolescent Psychiatry [AACAP], and the American Academy of Addiction Psychiatry, to name a few). Involvement in smaller, more intimate organizations has been of tremendous benefit to most successful academicians. The environment at smaller meetings and the opportunities for involvement on committees are especially appropriate for the special career development and mentoring needs of junior faculty and residents. Many organizations have mentoring programs designed for just this purpose; investigate these opportunities, get involved, and make yourself known in at least one of the smaller organizations.

Some of the criteria for appointment and promotion relate to your involvement in outside activities and professional service, as well as letters of recommendation from other psychiatrists who know you. One of the most important ways to meet and get to know other academic psychiatrists is to go to meetings, give presentations, serve on committees, and generally get to know the characters of the organizations.

### Applying for Fellowships and Awards

Gaining recognition through fellowships (e.g., for travel or to serve on a committee or board) and awards is an extremely valuable strategy used by successful academic psychiatrists (Roberts et al. 1999). Become aware

| TABLE 2–1. | Sample recipe for success |
|---|---|
| Year | Activities and priorities |
| PGY1 | • Choose a mentor (preferably two or more). Meet regularly; stay in touch.<br>• Read as much as possible.<br>• Consider several possible research/teaching/administrative projects to start on during PGY2 year.<br>• Try to write at least a literature review. |
| PGY2 | • Write a research protocol/curricular plan/other project plan; file institutional review board submission (if applicable), write a literature review.<br>• Start a project.<br>• Attend seminars when possible in your research mentor's lab or division.<br>• Join applicable committees and get involved. Find ways to formalize/operationalize teaching experiences.<br>• Apply for national fellowships through the American Psychiatric Association (APA) and other organizations. Network! |
| PGY3–PGY4 | • Write up research results/give presentation(s)/present curriculum plan/project.<br>• Collaborate, if possible, on data-based papers with senior faculty.<br>• Begin looking into fellowships (clinical, research, and administrative).<br>• Continue to gain teaching and administrative experiences.<br>• Apply for national fellowships/awards through APA and other organizations.<br>• Develop mentoring relationships with senior faculty outside of your own institution (network). |
| Fellowship year(s) | • Write research grant/apply for funding for academic project(s).<br>• Apply for national fellowships through APA and other organizations.<br>• Continue and intensify networking activities. |

of the available fellowships and awards, and let your department chair or residency training director know that you would be honored to be nominated for appropriate ones. A list of Web sites of psychiatric organizations appears at the end of this chapter.

## Professional Service

As a resident, you can make important contributions to professional organizations. The main requirement for making a contribution is the willingness to offer your time and hard work. Following through on a commitment will go a long way toward establishing your credibility. Working long distance (thank goodness for e-mail) on projects for committees is an excellent way to get to know other academic psychiatrists. Many of the current leaders in academic psychiatry began their careers in organizations in this way.

Although networking is covered elsewhere in this book (see Chapter 27), we would simply note that paying attention to networking early in your career is an extremely valuable investment; even more important, friendships and mentoring relationships develop out of these opportunities that last a lifetime.

## KEY CONCEPTS AND DEFINITIONS

**Mentor:** Works collaboratively and supportively with mentee to develop academic career goals. Sets realistic expectations, provides constructive feedback, helps mentee establish own goals, timelines, and priorities. Respects confidentiality.

**Mentee:** Works collaboratively and actively with mentor on career development. Respects accountability, offers details, explains behaviors and choices, expresses concerns, seeks feedback, and accepts feedback nondefensively.

**Trust:** A key ingredient in the mentor-mentee relationship. Establish it early on and do not break trust.

**Accountability:** Your mentor(s) need to know that you will follow through and complete projects in a timely, thorough, and conscientious manner. Your early attention to being accountable is crucial to your later success.

**Professional organizations:** Critical to your ultimate success in academic psychiatry, joining and participating actively in professional organizations will be fulfilling and will enable you to make professional contacts, not to mention lasting friendships.

**TABLE 2–2.** Sample menus for success, by academic orientation

| Academic orientation | Personal temperament and preferred working conditions | Skills to practice during residency (in addition to excellent clinical training) |
|---|---|---|
| The researcher | Enjoys working alone *and* in teams<br>Tolerates ambiguity<br>Can enjoy the writing process<br>Enjoys the creative process | Finding and working with mentors<br>Research and writing<br>Giving presentations<br>Teaching<br>Administrative skills<br>Statistics |
| The clinician-educator | Enjoys helping others' careers develop (e.g., students, residents)<br>Enjoys clinical work<br>Loves teaching and mentoring | Teaching residents and medical students<br>Administrative skills (e.g., giving feedback) |
| The administrator | Enjoys challenge of problem-solving<br>Enjoys team-building<br>Tolerates ambiguity<br>Enjoys working in "systems" and organizations | Managing others (e.g., by working as a Chief Resident)<br>Teaching<br>Serving on committees both within own institution and in national organizations |
| Combination of several academic orientations | Enjoys multiple processes/combinations of above; wants to combine various aspects of above in academic career | All of the above (who needs sleep?) |

## SMART STRATEGIES

- *Ask around about potential mentors* (e.g., fellows or junior faculty who have had mentors in the department), specifically inquiring about their strengths, limitations, or blind spots. Realize that different mentors will operate in very different ways and that not everyone's style will mesh perfectly with your own. Try to find a good fit. Also, it will be useful to identify at least two mentors—for balance, for exposure to more than one research area, and to gain a better understanding of how different people approach research, teaching, and administrative tasks.

- *Read and write!* Reading and writing cannot be overemphasized. The only way to get better at writing is to write. *Writing With Power* (Elbow 1998) is a fun, exciting book about writing (it is not focused on scientific writing, but the strategies for warming up and practicing writing are useful for anyone who must write). Writing is a crucial and large component of many successful faculty members' careers. You *can* improve your writing skills, contrary to what some believe, but it takes work and patience. A good place to start is to read more; read outside of psychiatry as well, but also familiarize yourself with the research literature. Read a variety of articles to learn about the structure and style of different kinds of scientific writing. Also, gain practice by offering to write literature reviews, helping whenever possible with data-based reports, and learning to review submitted manuscripts (Roberts et al. 2004).

- *Consider doing a research or administrative fellowship.* A fellowship provides the "protected" time that many junior faculty members need to develop a research plan, write initial grants, and publish. Many M.D.s feel that spending more time in training is a financial sacrifice. Consider, however, that this financial sacrifice for 1–2 years of fellowship may be offset by generous loan repayment programs (see the National Institutes of Health Web site at http://www. nih.gov) and can be viewed as an investment in your future, just as medical school and residency were.

- *Learn about and practice statistics.* Often this is a weak spot for M.D.s who choose to do research, because most have had very little statistics training. Try to take or audit a statistics course, arrange for a private tutorial with someone more experienced, or at the very least read a statistics text or two. There are some excellent, easy-to-read books that can serve as good starting points (e.g., *PDQ Statistics* by Norman and Streiner [1999]). You can also get practice analyzing datasets by asking your faculty mentors if they have data on which you could do some kind of secondary analysis. Finally, Web-based courses in statistics are available.

- *Practice speaking.* Give talks to medical students or junior residents. Most course organizers will be thrilled to have you offer to teach a session. Such activity forces you to gather and synthesize information (it is best to make your own slides rather than borrow someone else's) and to gain practice in public speaking. Many people avoid public speaking out of fear and anxiety, but it *does* get easier as you gain practice and confidence.

- *Look for specific mentoring opportunities* sponsored by local or national professional organizations, such as APA, AACAP, and AADPRT (to name just a few; many other organizations also sponsor mentoring programs). By joining and actively participating in organizations, you will meet new mentors, colleagues, and friends. You will also gain recognition as a resident who is already enthusiastic about academic psychiatry and is making contributions. If possible, join a committee and help with a project. Almost uniformly, committee chairs are delighted when people offer to help; use this to your advantage, but also make sure to follow through on commitments.

## QUESTIONS TO DISCUSS WITH A MENTOR OR COLLEAGUE

1. What were the most useful strategies for you as you worked your way to where you are today? (i.e., request tips for success)
2. Are there any things you would have done differently? Why?
3. Can you recommend other people I should meet with or talk to? Can you introduce me to _____ (i.e., ask for introductions to other people)?
4. What organizations and committees have been the most interesting to you? Which have been the most beneficial to your professional development?

## REFERENCES

Cohen NH: The Mentee's Guide to Mentoring. Amherst, MA, Human Resource Development Press, 1999

Elbow P: Writing With Power, 2nd Edition. New York, Oxford University Press, 1998

Norman GR, Streiner DL: PDQ Statistics, 2nd Edition. Hamilton, Ontario, BC Decker, 1999

Roberts LW, Warner TD, Horwitz R, et al: Honorary fellowship awards and professional development in psychiatry. Acad Psychiatry 23:210–221, 1999

Roberts LW, Coverdale J, Edenharder K, et al: How to review a manuscript: a "down-to-earth" approach. Acad Psychiatry 28:81–87, 2004

## ADDITIONAL RESOURCES

Below is a sampling of useful Web sites and phone numbers for residents interested in an academic career.

**Fellowship information:**

- American Psychiatric Association information for residents (several fellowships available):
  http://www.psych.org/edu/res_fellows/index.cfm
- American Academy of Child and Adolescent Psychiatry (numerous fellowships available):
  http://www.aacap.org/training/medRes/index.htm
- American Association for Geriatric Psychiatry:
  http://www.aagpgpa.org/prof/stones.asp
  Stepping Stones Program for Psychiatry Residents:
  http://www.aagpgpa.org/prof/fellows.asp
  AAGP Fellowship Program in Geriatric Psychiatry
- American Association of Directors of Psychiatric Residency Training information for residents (several fellowships available):
  http://www.aadprt.org/aadprt/fellowships.aspx
- American College of Psychiatrists (PRITE and Child PRITE Fellowships): Phone (510) 704–8020

**Professional organizations/journals:**

- *Academic Psychiatry*: http://ap.psychiatryonline.org
- Association for Academic Psychiatry:
  http://www.hsc.wvu.edu/aap
- American Academy of Addiction Psychiatry:
  http://www.aaap.org/membership/resident.html
- American Association for Emergency Psychiatry:
  http://www.emergencypsychiatry.org
- Group for the Advancement of Psychiatry:
  http://www.groupadpsych.org
- American Psychoanalytic Association:
  http://apsa.org/ctf/fellowship/index.htm
- Academy of Psychosomatic Medicine: http://www.apm.org
- American College of Neuropsychopharmacology:
  http://www.acnp.org
- Indo-American Psychiatric Association: http://www.myiapa.org
- Association of Women Psychiatrists: Phone (972) 686–6522
- American Academy of Psychiatry and the Law: Phone (800) 331–1389

# Strategies for Women, Minorities, and Other Underrepresented Faculty

Russell F. Lim, M.D.

Annelle B. Primm, M.D., M.P.H.

Donald M. Hilty, M.D.

This chapter focuses on career advice for early career psychiatrists who belong to underrepresented groups, such as women, ethnic minorities, and gay, lesbian, bisexual, and transgender (GLBT) psychiatrists who face additional challenges as academic faculty. The current status of underrepresented groups will be discussed, as well as strategies for success and pitfalls to avoid. The advice given in this chapter is intended for residents, specifically second-year residents, but it is applicable at any stage in one's career. Clearly, the earlier you get started, the faster and farther you can advance in your academic career. Special issues for underrepresented faculty include the importance of mentorship and networking, prioritization, and seeking out programs specific for that particular group.

## BACKGROUND INFORMATION

According to the Association of American Medical Colleges (AAMC) and the American Medical Association (AMA), ethnic minorities and women are underrepresented in academic departments of psychiatry, particularly in the senior faculty rank (American Association of Medical Colleges 2004; American Medical Association 2004). This phenomenon is often referred to as the "glass ceiling" (see Table 3–1). Faculty members of underrepresented groups are likely to be the only representative (or one of just a few) of their group at an institution, and there is concern that they may not be afforded the status and recognition of the mainstream members of the faculty. The lack of representation and role models is self-replicating and creates a vicious cycle; because medical students or psychiatric residents do not find faculty of similar backgrounds in the specialty of their interest, they may be less likely to go into psychiatry or academic psychiatry. Members of underrepresented groups may have greater difficulty getting jobs, finding collaborators, and getting promoted because of their isolation from the majority. The early career psychiatrist from a minority or underrepresented group has to create his or her own support groups, from within and outside the institution, and network for success.

## CAREER ADVICE

### Key Concepts

**Find a mentor:** Find someone who does things that you would like to do, and ask to join him or her on a project. Meet with that person regularly; while the person does not have to be a faculty member at your institution, it will be easier to meet if that is the case. Do not limit mentors to only persons of your underrepresented group, because that will limit your choices. See Table 3–2 for professional organizations, and see also the section "Questions to Discuss With a Mentor or Colleague" at the end of this chapter (see Chapter 26 for more on mentoring).

**Train:** Apply for underrepresented group–oriented fellowship, training, and grant opportunities. Identify and be aggressive about availing yourself of opportunities (e.g., master's of business administration, public health, federal grant minority supplements, loan repayments, fellowships, and National Institute of Mental Health [NIMH]– and AAMC-sponsored training) on grant writing and career development.

**Network:** Join the American Psychiatric Association (APA), and attend council meetings of your district branch by volunteering to be on a committee. You will meet many local members, as well as be kept aware of current issues involving your profession. Visibility is critical for under-

**TABLE 3–1.** Percentage of the U.S. population and medical school faculty and distribution of selected faculty by ethnicity, gender, and rank

| | Black | Asian | Hispanic | Native American | Caucasian | Male | Female |
|---|---|---|---|---|---|---|---|
| General population, 2000 | 12.3 | 3.7 | 12.5 | 0.9 | 75.1 | 49.1 | 50.9 |
| Medical school faculty, 2003 | 3.1 | 11.9 | 3.9 | 0.1 | 75.2 | 69 | 31 |
| Psychiatry faculty, 2003 | 3.4 | 7.2 | 4.1 | 0.2 | 78.5 | 62 | 38 |
| **Distribution among selected ranks** | | | | | | | |
| Medical school faculty, 2003 | | | | | | | |
| Professor | 9 | 14 | 16 | 21 | 28 | 30.3 | 11 |
| Associate professor | 17 | 17 | 18 | 17 | 23 | 23.3 | 18.6 |
| Assistant professor | 54 | 52 | 50 | 52 | 38 | 37 | 50 |
| Clinical instructor | 18 | 6 | 14 | 14 | 10 | 8.3 | 17.9 |
| Other | 2 | 4 | 2 | 3 | 2 | 1.1 | 2.5 |
| Psychiatry faculty, 2003 | | | | | | | |
| Professor | 12 | 15 | 20 | 33 | 28 | 26 | 8 |
| Associate professor | 16 | 16 | 15 | 11 | 24 | 23 | 16 |
| Assistant professor | 49 | 54 | 50 | 33 | 38 | 40 | 54 |
| Clinical instructor | 21 | 14 | 13 | 22 | 9 | 10 | 20 |
| Other | 2 | 1 | 3 | 0 | 2 | 2 | 3 |

*Source.* American Medical Association 2003; Association of American Medical Colleges 2004; U.S. Census 2004.

---

**TABLE 3–2.**   Professional groups for academics

---

**General**

American Medical Association (AMA) Minority Affairs Consortium,
http://www.ama-assn.org/ama/pub/category/20.html

American Psychiatric Association (APA) Office of Minority and
National Affairs, Council of Mental Health and Health Disparities,
Interest Groups, Assembly Committee of Underrepresented Groups,
and District Branches, http://www.psych.org/mem_groups

**Education-oriented groups**

American Association of Directors of Psychiatric Residency Training
(AADPRT), http://www.aadprt.org

Association for Academic Psychiatry (AAP),
http://www.hsc.wvu.edu/aap

Association of Directors of American Medical Student Education
Programs (ADMSEP), http://www.admsep.org

**Underrepresented groups**

American Society of Hispanic Psychiatrists (ASHP),
Javier I. Escobar M.D., President, escobaja@umdnj.edu

Asian Pacific American Medical Student Association (APAMSA),
http://www.apamsa.org

Association of American Indian Physicians (AAIP),
http://www.aaip.com

Association of Chinese-American Psychiatrists (ACAP),
Edmond Hsin-Tung Pi, M.D., edpi@usc.edu

Association of Gay and Lesbian, Psychiatrists (AGLP),
http://www.aglp.org

Association of Korean-American Psychiatrists (AKAP),
David Rue, M.D., drue@sutterhealth.org

Association of Women Psychiatrists (AWP),
http://www.womenpsych .org

Black Psychiatrists of America, 2730 Adeline St.,
Oakland, CA 94607

Indo-American Psychiatric Association (IAPA),
http://www.myiapa.org/index.html

National Medical Association (NMA), Psychiatry Section,
http://www.nmanet.org

Pakistani Psychiatrists Association of North America (PPANA),
Zahid Imran, M.D., Zimran4649@aol.com

Philippine Psychiatrists of America (PPA),
http://www.PPA-online.org

---

**TABLE 3–2.** Professional groups for academics *(continued)*

---

**Subspecialty groups**

   American Association of Community Psychiatrists (AACP),
      Diversity Committee, http://www.communitypsychiatry.org

   Society for the Study of Culture and Psychiatry (SSPC),
      James K. Boehnlein, M.D., james.boehnlein@med.va.gov

**International associations**

   Pacific Rim College of Psychiatry (PRCP),
      http://www.prcp.org

   World Psychiatric Association (WPA) Section on Transcultural
      Psychiatry, http://www.wpanet.org/home.html

**Referral-only group**

   Group for the Advancement of Psychiatry (GAP) Cultural Psychiatry
      Committee, http://www.groupadpsych.org

---

represented groups, and you can bring up issues pertinent to your group—you could even start your own committee (e.g., a diversity committee, a GLBT committee). Joining national organizations is also important, and there are many organizations focused on education, clinical care, research, and administration that could use input on diversity and could provide the early career academic psychiatrist with a broad-based support system that will come in handy at promotion time for extramural letters (see Table 3–2), as well as help to break the glass ceiling later.

**Prioritize:** Avoid succumbing to undue pressures to "represent the race (or group)" with citizenship activities that can require major time investment and jeopardize academic advancement through conflict of commitment. Keep in mind that both your presence and your absence are noted. In other words, when you are a member of an underrepresented group, you tend to stand out from the crowd. This can be good and bad, as you can be singled out to represent underrepresented issues. Remember that your presence as a member of an underrepresented group is an asset—sometimes this can bring funds to your department through supplements, grants, and fellowships. To avoid gaining a reputation for being unreliable, avoid overcommitment.

**Present your work:** Think about your clinical work, research, or teaching, and then prepare a presentation for local, regional, and national meetings. You may have to package it with other similar programs from different parts of the country for a national meeting. If you can, add an evaluation component and think about publishing in an appropriate journal.

**Publish, publish, publish:** If you are doing great work and no one knows about it, it won't make a major difference in how psychiatry is practiced or taught and you won't get promoted as faculty. Focus your energies and convert your presentations as much as possible into publications for peer-reviewed journals. In doing so, you can support the development of other minorities through collaboration and mentorship (see Chapters 21 and 22).

**Volunteer:** Get involved in your department. Get some experience with being on a committee or being in charge of one. You will need to develop a group of supporters and collaborators.

**Develop a mission:** The mission for one author (R.F.L.) was "to improve the quality of care for ethnic minority patients by first becoming knowledgeable, then teaching others, then creating models for others to follow."

**Get protected time:** And use it wisely (see Chapter 8). Also get time off for meetings that help you and the department on topics related to diversity rather than automatically using vacation; travel funds may be possible.

**Be a mentor:** Be a mentor for underrepresented residents and medical students (see Chapter 26). Offer to supervise them in clinical work and research, and encourage them to apply for minority fellowships from APA's Program for Minority Research Training in Psychiatry (PMRTP), the American Psychiatric Institute for Research and Education (APIRE), the U.S. Substance Abuse and Mental Health Services Administration (SAMHSA), AstraZeneca, Bristol-Myers Squibb, Janssen, and Glaxo-SmithKline. Help them network locally, regionally, and nationally, and encourage them to volunteer for teaching and leadership positions, such as chief resident. Finally, encourage them to consider a postgraduate fellowship in an area of interest, such as community psychiatry, substance abuse, child and adolescent psychiatry, psychosomatic medicine (consultation-liaison), forensics, or administrative psychiatry.

## ADVICE SPECIFIC TO WOMEN

In addition to the responsibilities listed above, women must also prioritize the competing demands of career and family—while recognizing that one cannot meet all demands because these two aspects of their lives may be at differing stages of development. It helps to have one's clinical assignment match one's research interest for the sake of efficiency, and female faculty members also need to know when to turn down less important opportunities that may demand time away from work and family, such as social committee work (although some committee work may be worth the time). While one is caring for young children, creativity may be necessary to meet academic career goals, for example through part-time or shared positions and time in academic series that do not have an "up or out" requirement.

Academic environments tend to be competitive, yet if a woman were to show the aggressiveness of a man, instead of what some believe should be her more natural instinct to work cooperatively, it might not be accepted in the same way. Mentorship and networking are even more critical to women faculty, who often feel shut out of the "old boy network." Dressing well is important, as is learning how to give a clear presentation. Relationships within the academic environment need to be handled carefully (e.g., avoiding romantic involvements with trainees and faculty, and being discreet with colleagues). Discretion is also important when dealing with child care issues during the 9 A.M.–5 P.M. working time (Leibenluft 1999).

## ADVICE SPECIFIC TO ETHNIC MINORITIES

Members of minority groups have to prove themselves to be competent, to dispel the stereotype that they are not as good as mainstream, Caucasian psychiatrists. The basis of this stereotype is that the faculty member was hired because of his or her group membership rather than qualifications. Pursuing an interest in minority mental health could result in marginalization if the research does not contain comparisons to Caucasian groups, whereas pursuing a culture-neutral interest may be seen as selling out. Minority faculty members who have an interest in research with minority groups may need to find collaborators at other institutions that have large enough minority populations to make their research statistically significant. Because racism is ubiquitous and often institutionalized, the minority early career psychiatrist should not take racial slights personally and should use them as opportunities to educate and enlighten colleagues about these issues (Darley et al. 2003).

## ADVICE SPECIFIC TO GLBT PSYCHIATRISTS

Unlike women and ethnic minorities, GLBT academic psychiatrists can hide their identity as underrepresented clinicians if they choose to do so. Disclosing one's minority sexual orientation has benefits in that the individual may develop a specialization in GLBT issues, as well as help to integrate personal and professional identities. He or she may also become a mentor for younger trainees. Nevertheless, it is important to mention that there is often considerable prejudice against GLBT individuals in academia, similar to that found in society, particularly in nonurban areas (Lu et al. 1999).

## CASE EXAMPLES

Finally, we will discuss two case examples of diversity initiatives, one supported by a department of academic psychiatry, the other by a national grant. The University of California, Davis, Department of Psychiatry and Behavioral Sciences has had a Diversity Advisory Committee (DAC) for the last 5 years. The DAC has been successful in developing 4-year curricula in cultural competence and in religion and spirituality. The group provides mentorship and support for the minority faculty in the department, successfully nominates residents to become fellows in the APA Minority Fellowship Program, and recruits minority faculty to UC Davis. Key factors in the program's success are regular meetings, clearly defined priorities (e.g., education, mentorship, and recruitment), a critical mass of interested minority faculty and residents, a diverse patient population in the community, and leadership by a faculty well connected to national organizations.

Faculty development programs that include a focus on mentoring for women and other minority groups have been described in the literature (Gates et al. 2003; Wong et al. 2001; Parker 2002). Gates described a concerted effort to recruit faculty residents and medical students to work in the field of dentistry, stressed the concept of developing the "pipeline," and described the importance of creating an environment accepting of diversity, along with selection criteria to include membership of those in underrepresented groups.

Wong et al. (2001) described the National Center of Excellence in Women's Health Initiative. This program provided funding from the Office of Women's Health within the U.S. Department of Health and Human Services, which in 1998 created six Academic Centers of Excellence specializing in clinical service, education, outreach, research, and leadership for minority female faculty. Many of the centers had funding for research and others had built-in networking opportunities. These included mentorship, breakfast or lunch meetings, awards to recognize outstanding service, and training opportunities (e.g., workshops on teaching and research, leadership book clubs, and symposiums on faculty development). Finally, Parker (2002) suggested the development of a training workshop for faculty to learn how to mentor medical students with varying ethnic backgrounds.

In summary, being a member of an underrepresented group presents some challenges to having a successful academic career. However, there are strategies that can make the process a bit easier, and they include finding a mentor, networking, seeking out extra training, applying for fellowships pertaining to a particular underrepresented group, mentoring residents, and being productive by choosing a research and clinical focus that embraces one's identity and ideals.

## SMART STRATEGIES

- Seek multiple mentors that fit your "mission." They can be either inside or outside of your department—having more than one is a good idea.
- Get protected time and time to attend meetings that will benefit you and the department.
- Plan a track for yourself.
- Consider extra training: M.B.A., Ph.D., M.P.H., postgraduate fellowship, workshops (e.g., on how to write grants and write papers), and clinical training (e.g., group therapy certification, CBT, psychoanalysis, and Jungian analysis).
- Take advantage of your underrepresented status by applying for special funding, such as minority supplements or fellowships and training opportunities, from APA and other organizations.
- Use your unique background as a strength by teaching others about your group's similarities and differences to the mainstream.
- Join organizations that value your perspective.
- Invite colleagues from different institutions that share your values and culture.

## QUESTIONS TO DISCUSS WITH A MENTOR OR COLLEAGUE

1. What professional organizations should I join for my interests?
2. What professional meetings should I attend for my interests?
3. Who should I contact about further information about my interests?
4. For institutional mentors: What committees should I become involved in, either in the medical school, department, university, or local district branch of APA?
5. How do I maximize my time to get promoted, that is, get help with managing projects, such as grants or publications?

## REFERENCES

American Association of Medical Colleges: Minority Medical School Faculty Roster. Table 3: Rank and Race/Hispanic Origin. Available at: http://www.aamc.org/data/facultyroster/usmsf03/03table3.xls, and Table 20: Sex, Race/Hispanic Origin, Rank, and Department. Available at: http://www.aamc.org/data/facultyroster/usmsf03/03table20.xls. Accessed November 29, 2004.

American Medical Association: Womens Physician Congress. Table 8: Medical School Faculty Distribution by Gender and Rank, 2003. Available at: http://www.ama-assn.org/ama/pub/category/12919.html. Accessed December 5, 2004.

Darley JM, Zanna MP, Roediger HL (eds): The Compleat Academic: A Career Guide, 2nd Edition [see Jones JM, Ree E: "The Dialectics of Race: Academic Perils and Promises," pp 295–310; and Park DC, Nolen-Hoeksema S: "Women in Academia," pp. 311–328]. Washington, DC, American Psychological Association, 2003

Gates PE, Ganey JH, Brown MD: Building the minority faculty development pipeline. J Dent Educ 67:1034–1038, 2003

Leibenluft E: Women in academic psychiatry, in Handbook of Psychiatric Education and Faculty Development. Edited by Kay J, Silberman EK, Pessar L. Washington, DC, American Psychiatric Press, 1999, pp 95–107

Lu FG, Lee K, Prathikanti S: Minorities in academic psychiatry, in Handbook of Psychiatric Education and Faculty Development. Edited by Kay J, Silberman EK, Pessar L. Washington, DC, American Psychiatric Press, 1999, pp 109–123

Parker DL: A workshop on mentoring across gender and culture lines. Acad Med 77:461, 2002

U.S. Census: Census 2000: Briefs and Special Reports. Available at: http://www.census.gov/population/www/cen2000/briefs.html. Accessed December 13, 2004.

Wong EY, Bigby J, Kleinpeter M, et al: Promoting the advancement of minority women faculty in academic medicine: the National Centers of Excellence in Women's Health. J Womens Health Gend Based Med 10:541–550, 2001

## ADDITIONAL RESOURCES

Cabaj B, Stein T: Textbook of Homosexuality and Mental Health. Washington, DC, American Psychiatric Publishing, 1996

Group for the Advancement of Psychiatry: Cultural Assessment in Clinical Psychiatry. Washington, DC, American Psychiatric Publishing, 2002

Hays PA: Addressing Cultural Complexities in Practice. Washington, DC, American Psychological Association, 2001

Kay J, Silberman EK, Pessar L: Handbook of Psychiatric Education and Faculty Development. Washington, DC, American Psychiatric Press, 1999

Kleinman A: Rethinking Psychiatry. New York, The Free Press, 1988

Pinderhughes E: Understanding Race, Ethnicity, and Power: The Key to Efficacy on Clinical Practice. New York, The Free Press, 1989

Stotland N, Stewart D: Psychological Aspects of Women's Health Care: The Interface Between Psychiatry and Obstetrics and Gynecology, 2nd Edition. Washington, DC, American Psychiatric Publishing, 2001

Talbott JA, Hales RE: Textbook of Administrative Psychiatry: New Concepts for a Changing Behavioral Health System, 2nd Edition. Washington, DC, American Psychiatric Press, 2001

Tseng WS, Strelzer J: Culture and Psychotherapy: A Guide to Clinical Practice. Washington, DC, American Psychiatric Press, 2001

# CHAPTER 4

# Strategies for Psychologists and Other Health Professionals

Jerald Belitz, Ph.D.

Brad K. Grunert, Ph.D.

Laura Weiss Roberts, M.D., M.A.

First, the good news: a 1997 survey by the American Psychological Association (APA) identified 4,958 psychologists who work in U.S. medical schools or academic health centers; it was found that more than 50% are housed in psychiatry and behavioral sciences departments (Pate and Kohout 2004; Williams et al. 1998). This signifies a twofold increase from the 2,336 psychologists enumerated in 1978 (Hong and Leventhal 2004). The less-than-good news is that academic psychologists represent only 3% of full-time faculty in medical schools (Hong and Leventhal 2004). Taken together, these data suggest that the importance of psychologists to state-of-the-art clinical care is increasingly recognized but that this has not as yet translated into strong representation on medical school faculty. For these reasons, it is important for early career psychologists who serve in academic departments of psychiatry to approach their professional development and careers strategically.

Psychologists from a wide array of specialty areas (e.g., clinical, developmental, health, neuropsychological, and rehabilitation) are well integrated into academic departments of psychiatry. In general terms, while the practice of psychiatry is a medical discipline with strong emphasis on the biological basis of illness, the practice of psychology focuses on a learning paradigm for understanding—and treating—problematic behavior.

The inclusion of psychologists within academic psychiatry departments thus allows for a potentially rich and fruitful exchange between these disciplines. Each of the paradigms provides a complementary set of interventions that can greatly benefit patients, as evidenced in recent research that shows that utilizing *both* medication and cognitive-behavioral techniques in the treatment of depression greatly reduces symptoms and enhances resiliency.

Beyond patient care, psychologists, with their training and experience in scientific design and data analysis, assessments, evidence-based interventions, and the biopsychosocial components of development and behavior, are distinctively equipped to help their departments realize their missions of research and education. APA reports that psychologists primarily expend their time in these three general categories: research, 43%; clinical service, 31%; and education, 20% (Pate and Kohout 2004).

It is vital for an early career psychologist to recognize that achievement in academic medicine will be accomplished through the demonstration of psychology's contribution to the department (see Chapters 5, 10, 11, and 12). This is actualized by a process of partnering with professionals in other disciplines to help the department attain its specific goals (Hong and Leventhal 2004). Psychologists who recognize their department's unmet needs and then satisfy them will be valued and successful. Daugherty (1997) cautions that psychologists must relinquish a "supply side" orientation and replace it with a "demand side" approach. Then, when credibility and worth are established, the psychologist has the flexibility to introduce new ideas and personal goals.

## PROFESSIONAL ISSUES

Several academic tracks are available to psychologists: tenure; research; clinician-educator; nonacademic. Though there are psychologists who select a research track, most researchers are subsumed under the tenure track. In 1997, approximately 50% of the psychologists were in the tenure track, 40% were nontenure faculty, and only 6% were in nonacademic positions (Williams et al. 1998).

In recent years, medical schools have reserved the tenure track for faculty whose primary responsibilities involve research, teaching, and patient service. Promotion is determined by excellence in the first two domains and competence in the third; however, significant importance is placed on research productivity. An increasing number of faculty members are directed to the clinician-educator track in which promotion is determined by excellence in teaching and patient service and by competence in scholarship. Early career psychologists are encouraged to choose a department that allows them to match their strengths and interests with the department's needs.

The clinician-educator track is unique to academic health centers (AHCs) because of their reliance on physicians to train residents and provide patient care. This track has not always been available to psychologists or other nonphysicians. As an example, the Faculty Senate of the University of New Mexico (UNM) originally voted to create the clinician-educator track exclusively for physicians, allowing them the full rights of tenure-track faculty. Through the efforts of psychologists in the Department of Psychiatry, notably ones who had established their value to their department and the medical school, several deans and department chairs advocated for the inclusion of psychologists in the clinician-educator track. Consequently, the Faculty Senate voted to grant AHC doctoral-level professionals the opportunity to select the clinician-educator track. These same psychologists collaborated with deans and department chairs to grant psychologists membership into the medical staff with full voting rights. APA reports that 56% of AHC psychologists are members of their school's medical staff (Williams et al. 1998). Psychologists at UNM, like psychologists throughout the nation, do not have admitting privileges.

Psychologists will confront many professional problems. Physician mentors who appreciate the value of psychology are excellent sources of support and guidance. Senior colleagues and program directors who are esteemed for their accomplishments and insight lend credibility to psychologists through their advocacy. As a result of their support, psychologists are appointed to committees (e.g., Institutional Review Board, Biomedical Ethics Committee) and included in new projects (e.g., school-based programs or other community outreach plans) that are critical to the department or AHC. Until psychologists secure leadership positions in their respective departments, physician colleagues are essential for the advancement of important issues such as promotion and salary equity.

Perhaps the most profound challenge in academic psychiatry is the economic revision of behavioral health care systems, particularly the proliferation of managed care. As psychiatry departments and medical schools struggle to maintain fiscal solvency, resources become more restricted and professional value is, in large part, measured by financial criteria. Undoubtedly, the issue with the most potential to create conflict is prescriptive privileges for psychologists. This has become a divisive issue in American health care. Wise psychologists will consult and collaborate with mentors and colleagues and develop positive working relationships with their department chairs. Irrespective of one's personal position on the issue of psychologists' prescribing authority, it will be the strength of interpersonal and collegial relationships that will allow professionals to tolerate differing perspectives while maintaining good will and mutual respect.

This process of consultation and collaboration with mentors and colleagues is also important in educating departmental leaders and promotion review committees within the medical school. It is unlikely that either of these groups fully understands the nature of the training, curricula, or licensure and credentialing necessary to become a practicing psychologist. At this time, as the National Register of Health Service Providers in Psychology and the Association of State and Provincial Psychology Boards are working toward a national certificate of professional qualification in psychology to promote reciprocity of licensure, the educational process becomes paramount. Psychological training is rigorous and standardized, and it requires the mastery of key areas in order to pass the national examination required for licensure in virtually every state and province. By making departmental leaders and promotion review committees aware of the standards required to acquire practice privileges, psychologists can maximize their credibility with the medical profession.

## RESEARCH MISSION

Historically, psychologists were valued because of their capacity to secure grants, conduct empirical research, and generally advance a medical school's scientific goals (Carr and Benjamin 1997; Hong and Leventhal 2004). Productive researchers understand the needs of their departments, secure funding to support their work, and collaborate with interdisciplinary colleagues. These psychologists obtain grant funding that incorporates their interests, the department's goals, the local community's needs, and the funding agency's priorities. Grant funding engenders research publications, which produces prestige and revenue for the department (Carr and Benjamin 1997) (see Chapter 23).

Through their work as academic faculty members, psychologists can do much to contribute to the general body of scientific knowledge, to the scholarly endeavors of their colleagues, and to the research mission of their departments by collaborating on research projects. Psychologists typically receive rigorous training in scientific design, research methods, and quantitative analysis, and they have much to offer their psychiatrist colleagues who may have had relatively little exposure to these topics during traditional medical training. By being readily available for consultation and analysis of data, doctoral-level psychologists can facilitate both the ease and the quality of departmental research programs. Through the use of more complex research designs and analyses, subtle behavioral and medical interactions can be examined and defined. Moreover, interdisciplinary research may enlarge and enrich the set of scientific questions pursued as the integration of biological, psychosocial, and learning paradigms contribute to explanatory factors in behavioral abnormalities.

Topics for interdisciplinary exploration range from neuroimaging to psychosocial interventions, and over the past decade there has been an emerging imperative to integrate research with clinical practice. Psychologists are expected to develop evidence-based interventions and practice guidelines for specific diagnoses and populations. In an era of managed care and diminishing resources, researchers should investigate the differing treatment needs of acute and chronic diagnoses and factor in the variables of cost-effectiveness, cost benefit, and quality assessment (Droter 1997; Elliot and Klapow 1997; Tovian et al. 2003).

Very recently, there has been a concerted emphasis on research that encompasses biological and behavioral sciences in the understanding and treatment of all health issues. The Institute of Medicine (2001) has advised funding agencies to allocate resources into interdisciplinary studies that investigate the relationship of biological, psychological, behavioral, and social variables with health improvement and disease prevention. In 2003, the National Institutes of Health called for interdisciplinary research related to the biopsychosocial variables associated with illness and chronic disease (Hong and Leventhal 2004). The Institute of Medicine (2003) identified specific health problems that require substantial attention, including major depression, severe and persistent mental illness, tobacco dependency, diabetes, cancer pain, heart disease, and medication management. Belar (2004) indicates that all of these conditions have psychosocial and behavioral components that interact with prevention and treatment. Psychologists are primed to participate in research projects such as these.

## PATIENT CARE

Psychologists provide a range of clinical services that can be relegated to three categories: assessment, intervention, and consultation. Assessment skills differentiate psychologists from other behavioral health professionals: in addition to the administration of personality and cognitive batteries, psychologists conduct evaluations in specialty areas such as neuropsychology and forensics. As psychologists extend their services to other departments in an AHC, they will have occasion to appraise the psychosocial and behavioral variables related to adaptation to disease, pain management, readiness for transplantation, and other disease processes (Brown et al. 2002).

Interventions flow from clinical research. To sustain their value, psychologists need to apply evidence-based interventions to specific patient populations (e.g., chronically mentally ill patients) and specific diagnoses (e.g., depression). Unless psychologists demonstrate the utility of their practices, managed care corporations and budget-conscious administrators will demand the use of less expensive and less effective interventions. Such demands include the use of less-qualified clinicians, restrictions on the length and types of treatment, sole reliance on biological treatments, and the application of one standard of care for all patients (Carr and Benjamin 1997; Sanderson et al. 1997).

In his paper on developing a clinical practice, Margolis (1997) accentuates the necessity of understanding the consumer market and fiscal realities. Clinical services should meet the needs of the local community while not duplicating already existing services and should match the overt goals of the department or satisfy newly observed opportunities. A financial analysis that calculates the cost benefit, cost utility, and cost of compliance with regulatory agencies should be performed.

Psychologists are vital members of interdisciplinary teams that bring a biopsychosocial perspective to patient care throughout the AHC. Their expertise and sensitivity in sociocultural issues and contextual care can be applied to disease prevention and management—as in helping cardiac patients manage their stress and anger, for example.

Consultation and liaison services are core components of psychiatry departments. Psychologists are typically asked to consult with difficult patients, including those who have limited capacity to be their own decision-makers or who engage in suicidal behavior or self-harm, fail to comply with the medical regimen, or maladjust to their diagnosis. Brown et al. (2002) define liaison services as the provision of education to other health professionals. Liaison is an excellent mechanism by which to educate others about the role of psychology and to network with others who have common interests.

The initial task facing any psychologist or other health care provider when joining an academic department of psychiatry is to define one's expertise and to create a valued clinical niche among the faculty specialties. This task can be challenging, as the fields of psychology and psychiatry often employ different nomenclatures, use different explanatory paradigms, and apply different techniques for evaluation and treatment. It is often beneficial, therefore, for the psychologist faculty member to directly discuss these differences with his or her colleagues. Moreover, in many settings it may be important to serve as an ambassador for one's discipline by explaining the strengths it brings to the clinical care of patients, for example, or to the theoretical understanding of illness or maladaptive behavior. Finally, it is valuable to articulate the complementary (not contradictory) nature of the paradigms of medicine and psychology, finding common ground rather than points of contention.

The second task facing the new faculty member who is a psychologist and clinician-educator is to establish proficiency in clinical care. The most straightforward means of accomplishing this goal is to collaborate with faculty colleagues in the care of complex patients by using specialized skills. The treatment literature is replete with well-defined behavioral and cognitive-behavioral techniques to deal with issues regularly encountered by the psychiatrist. Salient examples include clinical care for 1) patients with anxiety or mood disorders; 2) patients with severe and treatment-resistant illnesses such as eating disorders, personality disorders, or addiction-related disorders; and 3) patients with significant treatment adherence issues, for example, medication management in the context of bipolar affective disorder. Through such efforts, the new faculty member who is a psychologist can rapidly establish a reputation for clinical excellence through collaboration.

A similar approach can be helpful when encountering physicians outside of the psychiatry department. Oftentimes these physicians are even less aware of the benefits of integrated behavioral medicine for their patients. Therefore, it is important that the faculty member educate physician colleagues as to the available resources for the treatment of their patients. Many studies suggest that a majority of office visits to primary care providers are the result of mental health–related issues. Such visits can be time-consuming and frustrating for physicians. By establishing an expertise and a willingness to assist physicians in the management of these mental health issues, the new faculty member can both lower their frustration level and facilitate care for their patients. Through collaboration with psychologists, physician colleagues can continue to perform the medical tasks and interventions that have led them to their fields and can also be content that their patients are obtaining the psychological help they require. Psychosocial interventions in behavioral health that have demonstrated value include AIDS compliance and prevention, diabetes, weight loss, presurgical screening and coping training, and pain management. Often it will be incumbent on the psychologist faculty member working in these areas to further educate nonpsychiatrist physician colleagues about the benefits of including their psychiatrist counterparts in the management of complex cases in order to ensure optimal clinical outcomes.

## EDUCATIONAL MISSION

Psychologists are indispensable to the education and training of medical students, residents in psychiatry and other specialties, nurses, physician assistants, psychologists, and other health professionals (Pate and Kohout 2004; Williams et al. 1998). Traditionally, psychologists are employed as behavioral health educators to share their knowledge on such topics as development through the lifespan, learning theories, personality theories, assessments, and clinical interventions.

The prominence of evidence-based research and practice affords psychologists many new teaching opportunities. With their appreciation of the relationship between research and practice, psychologists are prepared to teach empirically derived interventions and best-practice guidelines to behavioral health providers. As an example, psychologists are adept with cognitive-behavioral therapies and can instruct residents in the treatment of depression, anxiety, trauma, eating disorders, and substance abuse (Conrod et al. 2000; Friedman and Whisman 2004; Mischel 2004; Schmidt et al. 2003; Spangler et al. 2004).

At a health-educator summit, the Institute of Medicine recommended that health care professionals learn to deliver patient-centered care as members of interdisciplinary teams (Belar 2004; Institute of Medicine 2003). Daugherty (1997) entreats psychologists to teach health care providers from all disciplines and specialties to focus on the personal and interpersonal aspects of practice. One salient concern for providers is treatment and medication compliance—patient-centered care, with its employment of patient engagement, communication, and relationship building, enhancing patient involvement, and compliance with treatment. Other areas that require educational attention include death and dying, ethnic and cultural diversity, gender issues, and ethics (Belar 2004; Daugherty 1997; Elliot and Klapow 1997). Because of their experience in working collaboratively with other disciplines, psychologists have the skills to educate others about the subtleties of group dynamics, communication processes, power hierarchies, and conflict resolution (Belar 2004; King 2004).

Finally, psychologists present a paradigm that encompasses a biopsychosocial approach to physical and psychological health and illness. Patient-centered care accounts for the multiple factors that relate to disease, disability, disease prevention, well-being, and quality of life.

## SMART STRATEGIES

- Focus on the importance of integrating evidence-based psychosocial interventions with the biological interventions utilized in psychiatry.
- Focus on skills in research design and data analysis.
- Determine the unmet departmental needs that you can address in order to create a niche for yourself.
- Educate your chair and the rank and tenure committee on the training, expertise, and credentialing of psychologists.
- Serve as an ambassador for psychology as a discipline.
- Establish proficiency in clinical care focusing on evidence-based intervention, which demonstrates the scientist-practitioner model in which psychologists are trained.
- Educate nonpsychiatry physicians on the benefits of integrated behavioral medicine for their patients' care.
- Provide resident training in areas of expertise such as psychodiagnostic assessment and cognitive-behavioral therapy.

## QUESTIONS TO DISCUSS WITH A MENTOR OR COLLEAGUE

1. How can I present my skill set to other department members to facilitate an environment of acceptance and growth?
2. In what ways can I develop my own scholarly interests and support the scholarly commitments of my colleagues?
3. How can I contribute to the clinical services provided by the department?
4. What is the department's model for training residents and other behavioral health trainees?
5. What mechanisms are present to facilitate my professional development within the department? Within the medical school?
6. Who are the successful psychologist role models in the department? How have they attained success within the medical school environment?

## REFERENCES

Belar CD: The future of education and training in academic health centers. J Clin Psychol Med Settings 11:77–82, 2004

Brown RT, Freeman WS, Brown RA: The role of psychology in health care delivery. Professional Psychology: Research and Practice 33:536–545, 2002

Carr JE, Benjamin AH: The future of psychology in departments of psychiatry. J Clin Psychol Med Settings 4:143–153, 1997

Conrod PJ, Stewart SH, Pihl RO, et al: Efficacy of brief coping skills interventions that match different personality profiles of female substance abusers. Psychol Addict Behav 14:231–242, 2000

Daugherty SR: Report of the training group on education and training. J Clin Psychol Med Settings 4:13–22, 1997

Drotar D: Report of the working group on research. J Clin Psychol Med Settings 4:23–28, 1997

Elliott TR, Klapow JC: Training psychologists for a future in evolving health care delivery systems: building a better Boulder model. J Clin Psychol Med Settings 4:255–267, 1997

Friedman MA, Whisman MA: Implicit cognition and the maintenance and treatment of major depression. Cognitive and Behavioral Practice 11:168–177, 2004

Hong BA, Leventhal G: Partnerships with psychiatry and other clinical disciplines: a key to psychology's success in U.S. medical schools. J Clin Psychol Med Settings 11:135–140, 2004

Institute of Medicine: Health and Behavior: The Interplay of Biological, Behavioral, and Societal Influences. Washington, DC, National Academy Press, 2001

Institute of Medicine: Priority Areas for National Action: Transforming Health Care Quality. Washington, DC, National Academy Press, 2003

King CA: Psychologists in academic health settings: key contributions to dynamic interplay among research, clinical practice, and policy domains. J Clin Psychol Med Settings 11:83–90, 2004

Margolis RB: Building and maintaining clinical programs. J Clin Psychol Med Settings 4:35–40, 1997

Mischel W: Toward an integrative model for CBT: encompassing behavior, cognition, affect, and process. Behav Ther 35:185–203, 2004

Pate WE, Kohout J: Report of the 2003 Medical School/Academic Medical Psychologists Employment Survey. Washington, DC, American Psychological Association, 2004

Sanderson WC, Riley TR, Eshun S: Report of the working group on clinical services. J Clin Psychol Med Settings 4:5–12, 1997

Schmidt NB, McCreary BT, Trakowski JJ, et al: Effects of cognitive behavioral treatment on physical health status in patients with panic disorder. Behav Ther 34:49–64, 2003

Spangler DL, Baldwin SA, Agras WS: An examination of the mechanisms of action in cognitive behavioral therapy for bulimia nervosa. Behav Ther 35:537–560, 2004

Tovian SM, Rozensky RH, Sweet JJ: A decade of clinical psychology in medical settings: the short longer view. J Clin Psychol Med Settings 10:1–8, 2003

Williams S, Wicherski M, Kohout J: 1997 Employment Characteristics and Salaries of Medical School Psychologists. Washington, DC, American Psychological Association, 1998

## ADDITIONAL RESOURCES

Brems C, Lampman C, Johnson ME: Preparation of applicants for academic positions in psychology. Am Psychol 50:533–537, 1995

Hembree EA, Rauch SAM, Foa EB: Beyond the manual: the insider's guide to prolonged exposure therapy for PTSD. Cognitive and Behavioral Practice 10:22–29, 2003

# PART II

## Getting There…

# CHAPTER 5

# Preparing Your Curriculum Vitae

Deborah Simpson, Ph.D.

Curriculum vitae, personal statements, biosketches, dossiers, and resumes are used by professionals to communicate who they are and to highlight particular areas of expertise for a specific audience. Each document provides key information about a professional's background, skills, experiences, and personal qualities. Yet what is included, how it is displayed, and its length differ depending upon the author's purpose and the intended audience. Because the conventions around documenting and communicating experiences and expertise vary by country, this chapter will focus on a typical format for academic medicine within the United States.

## FRAMING YOUR LIFE'S COURSE AS A SCHOLAR

The English translation of the Latin word *vita* is "a life's course" (Aston University 2005). For an academic faculty member, the curriculum vitae (CV) should be a multipurpose document. The first goal of this chapter is to highlight how the CV can, through its digital format, allow a faculty member to maintain a detailed chronological and annotated master record of his or her academic life. This master file can then easily be reformatted to serve several specific goals including academic promotion, a National Institutes of Health (NIH) biosketch, and career planning. The second goal of this chapter, consistent with *vita* as a life course, is to encourage faculty to utilize the CV as an opportunity to portray their varied forms of scholarship, highlighting their achievements using recognized and expanded definitions of scholarship associated with education (Fincher et al. 2000;

**49**

Simpson et al. 2004) and community engagement (Maurana et al. 2001).

Creating and maintaining a CV that is an accurate portrayal of your academic career requires considerable time, effort, and emotional energy. New faculty members often start with a CV that is only a couple of pages long. But with diligence, these pages can soon be transformed into a document that highlights their accomplishments thematically, connecting the values and passions that led them to choose an academic career. The process of presenting one's themes through accomplishments makes putting together a CV a powerful experience. Hence, faculty members often comment that creating their CV is more work than writing a paper! Yet they also relish the task because it is rewarding to see what they've accomplished—to feel really good about that—and to see what they need to do next. As you approach the CV, consider it a teaching tool for two audiences: you and others. Its purpose is to teach who you are, what you value, and how your academic career and accomplishments are aligned by presenting evidence of scholarship.

## HOW TO PRESENT WHO YOU ARE VIA A CURRICULUM VITAE

In general, academic CVs, though weighted and formatted to align with the institution's mission, have four major sections:

1. Academic demographics: Personal information, academic and faculty ranks and positions, education/training, board certifications, licensures (as appropriate), military service, and any current or previous professional appointments or experiences.
2. Professional affiliations and leadership or service positions: Professional society memberships, including offices held and committee responsibilities.
3. Faculty roles and mission-associated activities: Typically includes research, education, clinical and community service, along with local leadership positions and service to college and community.
4. Evidence of scholarship as judged by peers: Bibliography (e.g., papers, book chapters, grants); endurable products (e.g., course syllabi, teaching evaluations); recognition by peers via selection or invitation (e.g., study sections, editorial boards, visiting professorships, presentations at national/regional meetings).

The appendix to this chapter presents a typical CV format for academic medicine. Simpson and Woodson (2005) offer an annotated example of a CV designed to demonstrate how, through the use of subheadings and brief explanations, the threads connecting disparate events creates a CV demonstrating one's professional life course (available at: http://www.mcw.edu/display/displayFile.asp?docid=1132andfilename=/User/dbrown/MCW_CV_Annonated_Final_WEB.pdf). Guidance about what to include and layout and formatting instructions are also provided.

CVs typically progress through several stages of development, as briefly outlined below. Allocate the time needed to ensure that your CV accurately and elegantly presents your academic career and life course.

- *Stage 1: Revising Your CV to Meet Institution-Specific Format*
  If the CV format is not already available electronically, ask a recently promoted colleague to forward an electronic copy. Not only will this provide you with a ready-made template, there may be inclusions that you can use with only minor editing.
- *Stage 2: The Great Archeological Dig*
  Major CV updates often require faculty to find all of the talks, papers, committees, courses taught, and other academic activities in which they have participated and add them to their CV in the required format. If regular updating is not feasible, then drop a note into a CV file folder with all the pertinent information so that all your information is accessible in a single location when it comes time to update. If there are CV "orphans" (i.e., activities, roles, products that have no apparent home in the CV), create an orphan category at the end of your CV to record these items.
- *Stage 3: Am I My CV? (Marcdante 2004)*
  Ask yourself, "What are the three or four areas or accomplishments in my career of which I am most proud? Most well-known? Which are aligned with my values and reasons for being in academic medicine?" Critically review your updated CV and revise it (within your institution's guidelines) so that those thematic areas emerge. Subheadings along with brief annotations or, if necessary, insertion of new major headers in appropriate sections of the CV can highlight your thematic life-course threads.
- *Stage 4: My Critical Colleagues Say...*
  The CV is the academic record of your career. Its ability to tell your academic life course is dependent on your ability to clearly and cogently define who you are and what threads connect your values and beliefs to your scholarly work. Ask a colleague who knows your work well and, if possible, another who has experience serving on a faculty promotion committee to review your CV and provide additions and revisions (be sure to ask your colleagues where to include

the CV orphans). Meet annually with your department chair to discuss your academic progress, and heed the advice provided because he or she is your advocate for academic advancement. If your department chair is relatively inexperienced at your institution or in academic medicine specifically, meet with a senior colleague to obtain an added perspective. As with any critique, you should a) thank your colleagues and b) consider their recommendations carefully prior to incorporating them into the CV.

- *Stage 5: First Impressions Leave Lasting Memories*
  Typos, grammatical errors, inaccurate or missing page numbers, layout inconsistencies, and other presentation flaws reflect poorly on the author. Be sure to have an editorial maven do a final proof of your CV to catch any errors.

- *Stage 6: Transforming the CV into an NIH Biosketch or Brief Narrative*
  There will be times where you will have to quickly communicate your academic career life course in formats that differ from that of the CV. If working on a grant, you may be asked to send in an NIH Biosketch. If you are a presenter at a conference, you may be asked to send a one- to two-paragraph narrative for inclusion in the conference program. Once your CV is updated and formatted, these requests are relatively easy to complete. The key step is to determine which CV inclusions are relevant to the specific topic, role, or expertise that you seek to communicate with the target audience (e.g., NIH reviewers, conference attendees). An example of a NIH Biosketch form can be found at: http://grants2.nih.gov/grants/funding/phs398/biosketchsample.pdf or in Chapter 23 of this book.

## A THREADED DISCUSSION OF ACCOMPLISHMENTS

The profession of psychiatry engages faculty whose expertise is broad and inclusive—from mental health, behavioral medicine, and community partnerships to the sciences associated with cognition, genetics, and neuropharmacology. As a result, these faculty members have an amazing array of goals, values, roles, responsibilities, and ways in which their contributions collectively advance knowledge that is essential to improving the lives of people with mental illness (Roberts 2005). As scholars, faculty members must provide evidence that their accomplishments have contributed to the field. Biosketches, CVs, and narratives provide an opportunity to visually and dynamically present a threaded discussion of accomplishments that are grounded in the values and beliefs of each faculty member's contributions to improving mental health through patient care, research, education, community or academic partnerships for health, leadership, and advocacy.

## KEY CONCEPTS AND DEFINITIONS

### Resume

- Audience: Tailored to employer typically in business (not academia).
- Purpose: A compelling and cogent document that focuses attention on an individual's strongest qualifications (e.g., experiences and skills) specific to a particular position or job category (Newhouse 1999).
- Length: Typically one to two pages.

### Curriculum vitae

- Audience: Academic (Reis 2000).
- Purpose: To provide a comprehensive, longitudinal record of the individual's expertise in a specific field highlighting education and training in the field, experience, leadership, scholarship, and other qualifications specific to the missions of academia (e.g., education, research, service) (Colorado College 2005; National Institutes of Health 2005; York University 2005).
- Length: Typically 5 or more pages at instructor-level appointment to 50 or more pages for senior faculty. (To view the transformation of a traditional academic CV to resume, go to http://chronicle.com/jobs/99/12/99120301c.htm.)

### Dossier

- Audience: Variable.
- Purpose: To provide a summary of accomplishments using multiple documents including resume or CV, examples of one's best works specific to the field, a cover letter, and letters of support. The specific inclusions vary, and there appears to be no clear consensus as to what they should be (Heiberger and Vick 2003).
- Length: Variable.

## QUESTIONS TO DISCUSS WITH A MENTOR OR COLLEAGUE

1. Can you look at my CV and give feedback?
2. Am I telling my academic story in a way that accurately portrays who I am through my accomplishments?

3. Looking at my academic record, what would you consider to be my strengths? Weaknesses?
4. Do you think I'm on track for promotion? If not, what do I need to do?
5. What resources are available within the department to help me reach some of my goals?

## REFERENCES

Aston University: Latin abbreviations and expression. Available at: http://www.aston.ac.uk/lss/external/latin.jsp. Accessed February 11, 2005.

Colorado College: Curriculum vitae. Available at: http://www.coloradocollege.edu/careercenter/Publications/Packets1999/3CurriculumVitae.asp. Accessed February 11, 2005.

Fincher R, Simpson D, Mennin S, et al: Scholarship in teaching: an imperative for the 21st century. Acad Med 75:887–894, 2000

Heiberger MM, Vick JM: Learning the lingo: Part II. July 3, 2003. Available at: http://chronicle.com/jobs/2003/07/2003070301c.htm. Accessed February 11, 2005.

Marcdante KM: Are you your CV? Presentation given at the Excellence in Clinical Education and Leadership—Faculty Development Program. Medical College of Wisconsin, March 2004

Maurana CA, Wolff M, Beck BJ, et al: Working with our communities: moving from service to scholarship in the health profession. Educ Health 14: 207–220, 2001

National Institutes of Health: Virtual career center. Available at: http://www.training.nih.gov/careers/careercenter/. Accessed February 11, 2005.

Newhouse M: From CV to resume. December 3, 1999. Available at: http://chronicle.com/jobs/99/12/99120301c.htm. Accessed February 11, 2005.

Reis R: The basic science of CV [Chronicle of Higher Education Web site]. March 31, 2000. Available at: http://chronicle.com/jobs/2000/03/2000033102c.htm. Accessed February 11, 2005.

Roberts L: Department of Psychiatry and Behavioral Medicine: A message of welcome. Available at: http://www.mcw.edu/display/router.asp?docid=173. Accessed February 19, 2005.

Simpson D, Hafler J, Brown D, et al: Documentation systems for educators seeking academic promotion in U.S. medical schools. Acad Med 79:783–790, 2004

Simpson D, Woodson CJ: Annotated academic CV. Available at: http://www.mcw.edu/display/displayFile.asp?docid=1132andfilename=/User/dbrown/MCW_CV_Annonated_Final_WEB.pdf. Accessed March 2, 2005.

York University: Preparing for an academic career path: writing CVs, an introduction. Available at: http://www.yorku.ca/carers/ma_phd/academic_writingcvs.html. Accessed February 11, 2005.

## ADDITIONAL RESOURCES

*The National Institutes of Health's Virtual Career Center includes useful links to sites containing specific strategies for exploring career options, important career skills, and a strong section on "The Job Search Process" that contains materials on CV preparation:*

http://www.training .nih.gov /careers/careercenter

*A model for an academic CV is available from the American College of Physicians Online Resident Career Counseling Center:*

http://www.acponline.org/counseling/letrescv.htm.

# APPENDIX 5-A

# CURRICULUM VITAE TEMPLATE FOR ACADEMIC MEDICINE

Name
Title
Department

1. Home Address:

2. Office Address:

3. Place of Birth:

4. Citizenship:

5. Education:
   mm/yyyy–mm/yyyy    Undergraduate...
   mm/yyyy–mm/yyyy    Medical degree...

6. Postgraduate Training and Fellowship Appointments:
   Clinical
   mm/yyyy–mm/yyyy    Residency...
   mm/yyyy–mm/yyyy    Fellowship...
   Education
   mm/yyyy-mm/yyyy    Certificate in Clinical Education...

7. Military Service:
   mm/yyyy–mm/yyyy    U.S. Medical Service

8. Faculty Appointments (include secondary appointments):
   mm/yyyy–mm/yyyy    Clinical Instructor...
   mm/yyyy–mm/yyyy    Assistant Professor...

9. Administrative Appointments:
   mm/yyyy–mm/yyyy    Division Chief...

10. Educational Administrative Positions:
    mm/yyyy–mm/yyyy    Director, Fellowship Training Program...
                       • Brief annotation of responsibilities, scope of work...
    mm/yyyy–mm/yyyy    Director, Multidisciplinary Program...

11. Hospital and Clinic Administrative Appointments:
    mm/yyyy–mm/yyyy    Director, Clinic...

12. Hospital Staff Privileges:
    mm/yyyy–mm/yyyy    Hospital name and address

13. Specialty Boards and Certification:

| Board certified | Issue date | Expiration |
|---|---|---|
| American Board of Psychiatry/Neurology | mm/yyyy | mm/yyyy |
| ABPN–Subspecialty | | |

| Certificates | Issued by | Issue date | Expiration |
|---|---|---|---|
| CPR | AHA | mm/yyyy | mm/yyyy |
| ACLS | AHA | mm/yyyy | mm/yyyy |

| Licensure | Number | Issue date | Expiration |
|---|---|---|---|
| State license | xxxxx | mm/dd/yyyy | mm/dd/yyyy |
| Other state licenses | xxxxx | mm/dd/yyyy | mm/dd/yyyy |

14. **Awards and Honors:**
    mm/yyyy   Phi Kappa Phi
    mm/yyyy   Alpha Omega Alpha
    mm/yyyy   Best Teaching Service Award
    - Brief annotation regarding how you were selected, by whom, for what

15. **Memberships in Professional and Honorary Societies:**
    Academic/Clinical
    mm/yyyy–mm/yyyy          Alpha Omega Alpha Medical Honor Society
      mm/yyyy–mm/yyyy          • Chapter President

    Education
    mm/yyyy–mm/yyyy          American Association of Directors of Psychiatry Residency Training
    mm/yyyy–mm/yyyy          AAMC—Group on Educational Affairs
      mm/yyyy–mm/yyyy          • Member—Section on Graduate Medical Education

16. **Editorial Boards/Invited Reviewer:**
    mm/yyyy–mm/yyyy   Reviewer, *Academic Psychiatry*
    mm/yyyy–mm/yyyy   Reviewer, *Teaching and Learning in Medicine*
    mm/yyyy–mm/yyyy   Member, Editorial Board, *Clinical Teacher*

17. **Regional/Local/Appointed Leadership and Committee Positions:**

18. **National Elected/Appointed Leadership and Committee Positions:**

19. **Research Grants, Contracts, Awards, Projects:**
    Peer Reviewed
    Title:
    Source:
    Principal Investigators:
    Role:          (as listed on the grant)
    Dates:
    Direct funds:
    Comments:

    Non-Peer Reviewed

20. **Invited Lectures/Workshops/Presentations/Site Visits:**
    International
    Author(s), title, meeting/event, location, and date (mm/yyyy–mm/yyyy)
    National
    Author(s), title, meeting/event, location, and date (mm/yyyy–mm/yyyy)
    Regional
    Author(s), title, meeting/event, location, and date (mm/yyyy–mm/yyyy)
    Local
    Author(s), title, meeting/event, location, and date (mm/yyyy–mm/yyyy)

21. **Peer-Reviewed Workshops/Presentations:**
    International
    Author(s), title, meeting/event, location, and date (mm/yyyy–mm/yyyy)
    National
    Author(s), title, meeting/event, location, and date (mm/yyyy–mm/yyyy)
    Regional
    Author(s), title, meeting/event, location, and date (mm/yyyy–mm/yyyy)
    Local
    Author(s), title, meeting/event, location, and date (mm/yyyy–mm/yyyy)

22. **Institutional Committees:**
    Education
    Research

23. **Institutional Teaching Activities:**
    Health Professions Undergraduate Students
    mm/yyyy–mm/yyyy
    Medical Student
    mm/yyyy–mm/yyyy
    mm/yyyy–mm/yyyy
    mm/yyyy–mm/yyyy
    Resident Education: Psychiatry
    mm/yyyy–mm/yyyy
    mm/yyyy–mm/yyyy
    Resident Education: Other Specialties
    mm/yyyy–mm/yyyy
    Fellow education
    mm/yyyy–mm/yyyy
    Other Health Care Professionals
    mm/yyyy–mm/yyyy
    Faculty Development
    mm/yyyy–mm/yyyy
    Continuing Medical Education
    mm/yyyy–mm/yyyy
    Community/Lay Public
    mm/yyyy–mm/yyyy
    mm/yyyy–mm/yyyy

24. **Students, Faculty, Residents, or Fellows Mentored:**

25. **Community Service Activities:**

26. **Programmatic Developments:**

27. **Continuing Medical Education:**

**BIBLIOGRAPHY:**

**Refereed Journal Publications/Original Papers:**

**Books, Chapters, and Reviews:**

**Editorials, Letters to Editor, Other:**

**Nonrefereed Journal Publications/Original Papers:**

**Abstracts—Peer Reviewed:**

**Video, Syllabi, or Other Teaching/Educational Material:**
Peer Reviewed
Non-Peer Reviewed

**Orphans (delete this section before submitting for high stakes)**

| | |
|---|---|
| mm/yyyy-mm/yyyy | Staff Physician, Community Mental Health Clinic for Elderly |
| | • Not-for-profit clinic located in Healthcare Care Shortage Area |
| mm/yyyy-mm/yyyy | Member, Quality Assurance Committee |
| mm/yyyy-mm/yyyy | Author, problem-based learning case; standardized patient case |

# CHAPTER 6

# Interviewing for an Academic Position

Richard H. Gibson, M.D.

Laura Weiss Roberts, M.D., M.A.

Interviewing for an academic position is a key milestone in the professional life of an early career psychiatrist. It is a collaborative process involving time, attention, energy, and iterative interactions that allow a candidate and an institution to adequately assess one another. The institution will want to understand the candidate's clinical strengths (experience, expertise, productivity), academic promise (teaching ability, research potential), and other important qualities such as leadership ability, attitude toward teamwork, communication skills, flexibility, and responsiveness. The candidate will want to learn whether the organization is stable and healthy, whether the mission and values of the institution are sound, whether the immediate work environment is positive and the workload is reasonable, and whether there is opportunity for advancement.

In the end, the most concrete—and the most critical—outcome of this process is, simply, a job. Does this job represent a good fit between the skills, expectations, and aspirations of both the candidate and the institution? Will this be a position that will ensure the candidate the highest likelihood of professional success and personal well-being? This chapter offers practical advice for the early career psychiatrist to help sort out the answers to these questions.

## PREPARING FOR THE PROCESS

It is critical to grasp the importance of interviewing and to prepare in earnest for the collaborative process that interviews represent. Searching for an academic post usually takes a full 6–12 months. For a position that begins in July, for example, the candidate should be looking and interviewing in the late summer or early fall of the previous year.

Before approaching a position, think about what your dream job would be. It is extremely helpful to write your thoughts down, preparing an extensive description of what you ideally would like to find. In this process, consider what are your "absolutes" and what are your "preferences" professionally; Table 6–1 includes suggestions for key factors to address in your thinking. It is also valuable to obtain feedback from your faculty, teachers, and mentors—people who know you and can give you meaningful advice about the contexts and expectations that will increase your chances for professional fulfillment. It is good to ask for guidance and candor, particularly related to your potential weaknesses as well as your strengths. Such exchanges will flow nicely into discussions with your supervisor about which academic institutions and settings may be a match for you.

During this time, it is helpful to begin talking with colleagues throughout the country and to begin systematically searching for information on various institutions. Even if you plan or hope to stay at your current institution, it is very important to know what other programs are like and to understand the national picture. It is valuable to reflect on issues such as climate, geography, community, and salary and their importance to you and your family. Plan on feeling a bit dissonant and stressed during this process of investigation, particularly if employment for a spouse and schools for children are considerations. This can be an exciting yet stressful time for dual-career couples and families as they discuss job transition and possible relocation ideas.

Other issues to consider when searching for information on programs include getting a sense of the medical school and the role, character, and prestige of the Department of Psychiatry within the college or university. Additionally, is the department eclectic in its commitments? Are there obvious areas of emphasis (i.e., psychoanalytic, biological)? What are the affiliated institutions like? Many Departments of Psychiatry are affiliated with publicly funded institutions (state and county hospitals, mental health centers, and veteran affairs hospitals). What are the various academic settings where junior faculty work? It is helpful to explore current areas of research by faculty at target institutions and to

---

**TABLE 6–1.**    Factors to consider in finding a dream job

---

- Type of setting (academic center, research institution, public institution)
- Division of labor between research, teaching, clinical work, and administrative duties
- Salary, benefits, full- or part-time status
- Location (climate, housing, schools, opportunities for spouse)
- Departmental support (mentoring, methodological expertise, funding, administrative support)

---

*Source.*    Adapted from Saha SA: "A Survival Guide for Generalist Physicians on Academic Fellowships, Part 2: Preparing for Transition to Junior Faculty." *Journal of General Internal Medicine* 14:750–755, 1999.

begin looking for collaborators and possible mentors? (The importance of mentorship is discussed in detail in Chapter 26.) Even at this very early stage in the data-gathering process, it is helpful to find out about state licensure requirements.

Ask your advisors for guidance at every step along the way. They may be willing to contact other institutions and to talk with colleagues to obtain information and to promote your candidacy. Although an institution may not be advertising an open position, many departments will work to create a position should they find a promising junior faculty member.

## JOB ANNOUNCEMENTS

You can now begin exploring job notices in professional journals and on-line postings and you may elect to get in touch with departments that seem especially interesting to you. When writing to inquire about positions, responding to an ad, or communicating with a search committee, it is crucial to compose a carefully written cover letter to accompany your curriculum vitae. This task should be taken very seriously because you are introducing yourself to this institution, and first impressions do in fact count. In the letter, briefly describe your interests and experience as well as your clinical, teaching, and research promise. Include an appropriate closing, indicating that you will follow up (Colorado College 2004; Duke University 2005). Attention to detail is important—proper spelling of the name and title of person you are writing to is a basic expectation (the letter should never be addressed "To Whom It May Concern"), and you should provide clear and accurate information on how you may be reached. The task of writing the letter should be effortful and should not be taken lightly—a clear, thoughtful cover letter is impressive and a great beginning to a relationship with a future employer and organization. One other housekeeping note: it is best if you send your letter both in hard copy (to be correctly formal) and electronically (to assist the recipient who may wish to forward the letter to others).

## STARTING THE CONVERSATION

Approximately a week later, follow up the letter and CV with a call to the department chair or chair of the Search Committee (see Chapter 4). Remember to be respectful, relatively formal, and considerate in all your verbal exchanges, especially to the secretarial staff. Be prepared for a brief chat over the phone and practice short responses to these likely questions: 1) tell me about your interest in us; 2) what is your area of research? and 3) what are your goals? Your responses should flow naturally, given all the work you have done prior to developing your vision of the ideal job. It would also be helpful to be complimentary to the institution and cite some specific strengths that you are aware of from your searching (both in your cover letter and in early interactions).

If you have made a positive impression, you may be contacted for several phone interviews by faculty. The goal of these interviews is to get some general impression of how well you might fit in with the department. At this stage, determine your point of contact, typically the department chair or a senior faculty member who can provide information and updates. Expect that each institution will do things a little differently. Be patient and do not personalize the inevitable frustration that occurs in communication, scheduling, and so on; this is a time for extreme flexibility.

## INTERVIEWS

If all goes well, you will be invited for a first interview visit. Typically, this visit will take place over the course of 1–2 days. It is generally anticipated that the department will cover travel and lodging expenses, but it is not always the case that they do so. It is not inappropriate to inquire tactfully about these matters.

Typically, you will be scheduled for a series of 30–60-minute individual interviews with various faculty members. Ideally, you should have input into who you meet based on your academic interests. It is important that you ask to have this input, and most departments will strive to accommodate your needs. If they do not, take that into consideration when making your final decision. Proper etiquette is that the department assumes responsibility for getting you to all of your appointments on time (arranging taxis, guides, etc.).

Plan to arrive the day before your interview begins. This gives you some time to get your bearings, have dinner with a colleague, and generally prepare. Interviewing tends to be physically and emotionally draining, so a good night's rest is critical.

People with whom to meet include faculty members in areas of research and education (not just in the Department of Psychiatry), representative junior faculty, the department administration, affiliate heads, program heads, the medical student and residency training coordinators, and the department chair (who will typically be one of the last interviewers). Be assured that many of these people will be dialoging behind the scenes as your visit proceeds.

Now is the time to implement all the listening and assessment skills you learned during residency. You are trying to determine the overall functioning of the department as a system and how it might work for you. Your questions should follow from these concerns. Examples of the topics that first-visit questions might cover include a description of the department's and institution's strengths and weaknesses; research areas and strengths; educational areas and strengths; positions available now and in the immediate future; communication within the department; the style and approach of the leadership; the promotion process; availability of mentoring; expectations concerning clinical time and protected time; efforts by the department and the institution to facilitate professional development and academic growth; compensation and patterns of financial stability within the department and institution; whether start-up resources are available for new faculty; and what infrastructure support (secretarial, typing, statistical) is available. It is especially important that as you go from interview to interview, you begin to make your own assessment of the morale. Would it be a fun place to work? Do people seem fulfilled and happy? Get a sense for people being on the same page on critical issues such as departmental mission, vision, and goals. What is the feel of the place? This may help you gain a sense of whether you would find a comfortable fit in the role.

Because interviewing is a two-way street, the faculty with whom you are meeting will be assessing you as you are them. You may be asked during this visit to give a "job talk" (a brief presentation on an area of academic accomplishment or interest). Find out who your audience will be and tailor your talk appropriately (for several resources on this topic, see Cordell 2005, Kroenke 1987, and Manuel 2000). Williams et al. (2005) suggest a useful format for thinking about how a search committee thinks. They outline the five Ws of the interview process:

1. *Why* do you want to come here?
2. *Where* do you expect to go academically in the next 5 years?
3. *Who* have you worked with? Who have been your colleagues?
4. *What* do you want to learn about our school? What do you expect from our school?
5. *When* will decisions be made? What happens next?

The interview with the department chair is often scheduled last. He or she will have had input (verbally, at least) from the majority of people with whom you have interviewed. At some point the department chair will want to hear from you on your overall sense of the department and what you think you can bring to the position. If you choose to broach the subject of your departmental criticisms or concerns, do so very tactfully; this is not the time to bring forward a litany of what you see as departmental weaknesses. However, if you wish to comment on potential areas for growth and niches where you can contribute (be genuine!), then go ahead (see Chapters 7 and 12).

You may find it helpful to jot brief notes immediately after this meeting. These notes will be invaluable, especially if you look at several positions within a brief time period. Finally, you should not leave before you have an idea of what happens next (when and how will you hear, etc.).

## SENSITIVE ISSUES IN INTERVIEWING

This may be a perfectly obvious point (and we hope it is), but it is absolutely essential to use good manners and to be formal and maintain appropriate boundaries during the interview process, even if it is at your home institution. Sadly, we still hear stories of candidates drinking too much at dinner, disrespecting departmental secretaries, spouting off provocative comments, or wearing jeans, shorts, or sandals. Such behaviors will cause the interviewers to wonder about the candidate's maturity and judgment. Use your common sense; ask your supervisor if etiquette is an area you should brush up on. It is better to hear this from your friend than from a no-longer future boss. Helpful literature can be found on the Web that goes into detail on issues such as behavior and conduct during interviewing (Alguire 2005; Career Recruitment Media 2005a, 2005b).

Candidates should also be aware of questions that are illegal (proscribed by federal, state, or local laws). For the employer, the focus of the questions and interview must be on what they need to know in order to decide whether the person can perform the functions of the job. Illegal questions often concern topics of family status, age, creed, pregnancy, race, or physical condition. Kaplan (2005) suggests three options for responding to an illegal question:

- *Answer the question.* You're free to do so, if you wish. However, if you choose to answer an illegal question, remember that you are giving information that isn't related to the job. In fact, you might be giving a "wrong" answer that could harm your chances of getting the job.
- *Refuse to answer the question,* which is well within your rights. Unfortunately, depending on how you phrase your refusal, you run the risk of appearing uncooperative or confrontational—hardly words an employer would use to describe the ideal candidate.
- *Examine the question for its intent* and respond with an answer as it might apply to the job. For example, it is illegal for the interviewer to ask, "Are you a U.S. citizen?" or "What country are you from?" However, you could respond with, "I am authorized to work in the United States." Similarly, let's say the interviewer asks, "Who is going to take care of your children when you have to travel for the job?" You might answer, "I can meet the travel and work schedule that this job requires."

Generally speaking, the interviewers will be well-meaning individuals without formal training in hiring and interviewing practices. Many of them may be more uncomfortable in this situation than you are. Consulting the literature will give you some familiarity with different types of interview settings and styles of questioning (e.g., team interviews, performance-based questions, stress interviews). Many faculty interviewers unknowingly pick up patterns of inquiry that mirror these styles. If you are comfortable with these styles, it will only strengthen the impression you give.

If you find you are being sexually harassed during an interview, tactfully bring the interview to a close. Report immediately what happened to the department chair or dean of the medical college. It would be best to write down your recollection of events.

## AFTER THE INTERVIEW AND THE SECOND VISIT

Follow up your visit with a letter. Written follow-ups range from letters and thank you cards to a strategic letter, which is recommended. A strategic follow-up letter conveys appreciation, re-articulates your interest, and covers one or two key themes for the position. Content will vary from letter to letter (i.e., letter to department chair vs. letter to potential colleague with whom you've interviewed). Brief thank you notes are appropriate for administrative staff.

If you've made a favorable impression, often you will be invited back for a second visit. You should accept only if you are interested. Before you go, try to obtain a draft job offer to discuss with your colleagues and supervisor.

The second visit is much more detail oriented. It is a time for focused discussion of concerns identified earlier and also an in-depth look at your clinical assignment. During the second visit, strive to begin clarifying as many issues as possible regarding the position, such as salary, benefits, specifics surrounding your academic appointment, time commitment expectations, office logistics, and departmental support structures; this will often involve negotiating (see Chapters 7 and 12).

In summary, the academic job interviewing process is a critical milestone in your professional and personal life. With thoughtful preparation, you will give yourself an excellent shot at finding a position that works for you.

## SMART STRATEGIES

As you are preparing for interviews, ask yourself the following questions:

- What type of academic position am I seeking?
- How would I prioritize the different components in my description of the ideal job?
- What is my academic timeline for information gathering, interviewing, and making a decision?
- What other personal elements are important to this decision (family and spousal considerations)?
- What institutions should I target in my search?
- What are my overall impressions of departmental morale, mission, and collegiality at each site?
- How would I make a decision if offered a position after or during my first visit?

## QUESTIONS TO DISCUSS WITH A MENTOR OR COLLEAGUE

1. Can you give me feedback on my description of my "dream job"?
2. What academic institutions might represent a good fit for me?
3. What strengths and weaknesses do I bring to an academic setting?

# REFERENCES

Alguire P: Tips for the first interview [American College of Physicians Web site]. Available at: http://www.acponline.org/counseling/tips.htm. Accessed February 11, 2005.

Career Recruitment Media, Inc.: Interviewing: dressing for the interview [Placement Manuals Online National Edition Web site]. Available at: http://www.placementmanual.com/interviewing/interviewing-06.html. Accessed February 11, 2005a.

Career Recruitment Media, Inc.: Interviewing: professional etiquette [Placement Manuals Online National Edition Web site]. Available at: http://www.placementmanual.com/interviewing/interviewing-08.html. Accessed February 11, 2005b.

Colorado College: Guide to cover letter development. Available at: http://www.coloradocollege.edu/careercenter/publications/pdfs/cover_letter_development.pdf. Accessed August 7, 2004.

Cordell WH: Preparing a presentation and developing speaking skills [Society for Academic Emergency Medicine Web site]. Available at: http://www.saem.org/publicat/chap8.htm. Accessed February 11, 2005.

Duke University: Career Center: The CV and Faculty Cover Letter. Available at: http://www.career.studentaffairs.duke.edu/grad/programs/insightscvletter.html. Accessed February 11, 2005.

Kaplan R: Handling illegal questions [Jobweb Web site]. Available at: http://www.jobweb.com/resources/library/Interviews/Handling_Illegal_46_02.htm. Accessed February 11, 2005.

Kroenke K: The 10-minute talk. Am J Med 83:329–330, 1987

Manuel D: Acing the academic job talk: Marincovich gives pointers. Available at: http://www.news-service.stanford.edu/news/2000/February9/jobtalk-29.html. Accessed August 16, 2004.

Saha SA: A survival guide for generalist physicians on academic fellowships, part 2: preparing for transition to junior faculty. J Gen Intern Med 14:750–755, 1999

Williams R: Interviewing for academic jobs [University of Michigan Web site]. Available at: http://www.cpp.umich.edu/students/gradservices/academic/intvtran1.htm. Accessed February 11, 2005.

# ADDITIONAL RESOURCES

Applegate WB: Career development in academic medicine. Am J Med 88:263–267, 1990

Fry R: Your First Interview. Franklin Lakes, NJ: Career Press, 2002

McCabe L, McCabe ERB: How to Succeed in Academics: Successful Career Management. San Diego, CA, Academic Press, 2000

Simon H: Obtaining a faculty position in academic emergency medicine. Pediatric Emergency Care 13:130–133, 1997

# CHAPTER 7

# Evaluating Your Contract/Letter of Offer

Andrew Norton, M.D.

Receiving your first contract or letter of offer is an important milestone for an early career psychiatrist. This document represents the culmination of the interview process in which an organization officially states its wishes to enter into an employment relationship with the recruited physician.

By the time the contract or letter of offer is in hand, your considerable work experience and an extensive interview process will have prepared you to carefully consider the position (see Chapter 6). You will have completed most of your postgraduate, residency, and fellowship training, during which time you will have had a significant number of opportunities to work with senior colleagues in an academic environment. Having gone through an extensive interview process, likely with site visits and first and second interviews at multiple academic institutions around the country, you will already know a lot about the environment in which you're contemplating working. You may also have explored nonacademic, private practice opportunities. Hopefully, you will have spent a significant amount of time thinking carefully about your life and career goals, discussing them with family and close professional colleagues (see Chapter 6). If you have wisely and carefully contemplated your career goals, used the interview process to compare and contrast employment situations and opportunities, and done some reading in the area of professional contracts, then you will be well prepared and confident in reviewing the contracts/letters of offer you receive. The aim of this chapter is to help prepare you for the task of evaluating and understanding key elements of the document you receive from a potential employer.

## BEFORE RECEIVING THE CONTRACT/LETTER OF OFFER

During your interview process, you should ask for the official employment handbook of the institution at which you are interviewing. These standard handbooks are available but often are not given to candidates until the time the contract/offer letter comes. Obtaining a handbook during the interview process will give you time to review elements of your official employment relationship with the institution, along with considerable background information that will be important in understanding various aspects of your contract/letter of offer.

Most candidates are told verbally that they are being offered a job and find that there is a slight lag between then and the arrival of the written contract/letter of offer. Strongly consider using this window of time to send a letter to your potential department chairman or division chief reflecting, in your words, what you think the job elements and expectations are. This represents an opportunity for you to communicate what you thought you heard as it relates to the job elements and expectations and what you think is most important. You should highlight the key deliverables that you expect to be covered in your written contract/letter of offer. Taking this proactive step will often shorten the negotiation process and bring clarity to key elements of the job opportunity.

## THE CONTRACT/LETTER OF OFFER

Many academic institutions draft a letter of offer, not a traditional contract. The legal difference is negligible, and for academic institutions that do not use formal contracts, a signed letter of offer will carry the weight of a formal contract.

The letter of offer is typically composed by the hiring department chairman or division chief with the assistance of the department's administrator. It outlines the key elements of the job but may lack the detail you will need to fully understand job expectations. Unfortunately, applicants often feel in a position of inferiority to the recruiting division chief or department chair, making them reticent to press for details—particularly if they are applying to their own institution, where they have worked in a trainee's role. Nevertheless, this is an opportunity to be sure that you have a clear understanding of all elements of the job. The clearer your understanding before taking the job, the fewer concerns and the less confusion you will experience at a later stage of your career at that institution.

Typically, your offer will have two main parts: 1) the letter of offer and 2) the official employment handbook including human resource policies and related documentation. Key aspects of the letter of offer include academic rank; terms of employment; job expectations; compensation; termination and severance agreements; and restrictive covenants (for a sample letter, please refer to the Appendix to this chapter).

## Components of the Letter of Offer

### Academic Rank

Academic rank will be assigned by the division chief or department chair and is typically not up for negotiation for an initial hire. However, the offer presents a good opportunity to understand the promotion criteria of the academic institution you're joining. Most have summary documents that can be obtained at this time.

### Terms of Employment

Most academic centers have self-renewing annual employment terms. Clarify that the employment is continuous and self-renewing based on a fixed term length or the faculty member's ongoing interest as well as performance.

### Job Expectations

This section of the offer will include general descriptions of your responsibilities, including

- Clinical activities
- Teaching
- Research
- Administrative duties
- Community service
- Academic service (e.g., membership on committees)

For each of these core elements of your academic career, you want to be focused on key components such as the proportion of your full-time equivalent position dedicated to each role, how you will be compensated for your efforts, and how your performance will be measured. Often not discussed are the lines of authority and the implications of job assignments. Clarify with your division chief or department chair who specifically is your superior and to whom you must account for your job responsibilities in each of these areas. Although most often you will be accountable to the division chief or department chair, be aware of co-management environments such as clinics that have medical directors; research laboratories; core laboratories that have directors; and hospital services in which responsibility is shared with hospital directors. Each of these could create confusion regarding time allocations, measurement of accountabilities, and resource allocations.

For those with a significant allocation of time to the clinical environment, pay particular attention to the specifics of the working environment. Although most of this will have been discussed during your visits, make a request that the details be written into the letter of offer. Question topics include what clinical resources will be made available (e.g., nonphysician clinical extenders), whether clinic overhead is linked to compensation, and how clinical compensation will be calculated (whether it is a relative value units–based method or related to fees and net reimbursement). Call coverage is critical and should be clearly defined. It's important to know what effects there would be with changes in your practice partners on your clinical workload, compensation and call coverage.

Compensation includes base salary, incentives, and bonuses. Be sure you understand the mechanisms by which incentives and bonuses are determined, timelines for payout, and who is in charge of setting the incentives and determining the metrics. Professional funds available for computers, work expenses, CME, and related expenses should be explained. National benchmarks for salaries and benefits can be obtained from national groups such as the Association of American Medical Colleges (AAMC) and the Medical Group Management Association (MGMA).

## Termination, Severance Agreements, and Restrictive Covenants

Many contracts and employment relationships include a process by which a nonrenewal or a termination process can take place outside of a grievance process. This would be used if a faculty member had performed adequately but was not felt to be a good fit for a long-term faculty position. Most academic centers have a 1-year, nonrenewal component in their contracts. As a result, most medical centers do not have severance agreements, although these can be negotiated in individual circumstances. Employment agreements typically are now applied to all new faculty. Employment agreements are used to protect the business interests of the hiring academic institution while the faculty member is employed or after the employment relationship ends. They typically have three components: a confidentiality provision, a nonsolicitation clause, and a restrictive covenant. The confidentiality provision prevents postemployment solicitation of other employees and/or patients, and the restrictive covenant outlines restrictions on postemployment competition with the academic center. Understanding these agreements in detail is critical, and most legal authorities feel that they are enforceable if reasonable.

## Employee Handbooks

Employee handbooks tend to be the clearest guide to the employment relationship at your academic center. The employee benefit package is typically best defined in these materials provided by the medical school's human resources department. This is key information to get in advance and review in detail. With the proper preparation, specific questions can be asked and answered during the interview process, but at a minimum these provisions should be reviewed after the interview and prior to signing the contract/letter of offer. Some basic elements:

- Health insurance
- Life insurance
- Long-term disability
- Malpractice insurance
- Vacation and sick time benefits
- Retirement plan, including times of vesting, etc.

Employer policies and procedures as they relate to such diverse issues as grievance and due process, Health Insurance Portability and Accountability Act (HIPAA) information and other confidentiality agreements, and codes of conduct or related professional behavioral policies are enclosed with these human resources materials and should be reviewed.

It is often these key elements of an employment relationship that are least understood by the department chair or chief who will be guiding you through the recruitment process. Department administrators and members of the central human resources office of the institution are excellent resources on the specifics of the employment relationship. Asking for a scheduled time with a human resources representative as part of your interview process will be helpful in your final review of your contract/letter of offer.

Finally, a few comments on whether to obtain legal advice. Contractual language may be nuanced. Terms like "at least" and "no less than" that imply a floor but no ceiling to work hours may allow unnecessary ambiguity. Lawyers will help with important clarifications and legal elements of the contract or letter of offer. When is it appropriate to hire a contract lawyer? It depends on the complexity and duration of the contract; on issues such as employment agreements that include restrictive covenants and control over intellectual property; and on the legal expertise and comfort of the physician.

## SMART STRATEGIES

- Do your homework. Learn about academic practices and the basic constructs of an academic career prior to any interviewing. Do site-specific preparation if at all possible.
- Categorize broad areas of employment for consideration (e.g., benefits, compensation, call coverage) and keep a comparison grid that allows you to look at the various opportunities in a systematic and organized way.
- When given a verbal offer, and prior to receiving your formal letter of offer, prepare and send a written summary of the job and its key elements *as you understand it*, which will help set a framework for the formal letter of offer and negotiations of key points.
- Spend time with the employee handbook and understand those key areas of basic employee benefits (e.g., health insurance, disability insurance, malpractice coverage).
- Don't be shy. Be willing to negotiate key elements and to ask for clarifications *in writing* of key elements such as compensation, distribution of work effort, call coverage, and bonus programs.
- The more you clarify before you sign, the less likely you'll have an issue after you've started your employment. Good academic candidates are rarely under time pressure to complete their negotiations once a verbal offer is made. Take the time to build a contract/letter of offer you're comfortable with.
- Avoid ambiguities. Contracts and letters of offer may lack precision. Get clarifications in writing before signing.

## QUESTIONS TO DISCUSS WITH A MENTOR OR COLLEAGUE

1. In retrospect, what were the key successes or regrets that you had in applying for and negotiating your first academic position?
2. What key element of the process would you recommend that I focus on?
3. What resources do you find most valuable in the process?
4. What is the one thing you wish you had known in advance of your first job search that you'd like me to know?

# APPENDIX 7–A
## SAMPLE LETTER OF OFFER

[Date]

Dear Dr. _____:

We are pleased to extend to you an offer of appointment to the full-time faculty of the _____ in the Department of Psychiatry, anticipated to commence on October 1, 200X.

Your appointment will be proposed at the rank of Assistant Professor. Policies governing faculty appointments are contained in the enclosed *Information for Faculty* handbook....

Your initial contributions to college and departmental missions in the areas of patient care, teaching, research, and administration/service will be as follows: _____.

*Patient care*: Your primary clinical assignment will be _____. In addition to this inpatient work, you will devote approximately six (6) hours per week to the Department's Consultation-Liaison (C/L) Program _____ _____ directed by _____. You will be expected to participate in the on-call rotation, with duties consistent with your team members. We anticipate this will be _____.

*Teaching*: In your role, you will be expected to participate in the multidisciplinary educational programs of the Department, to include _____ _____.

*Research*: In your role, you will be expected to collaborate with faculty involved in clinical trials and other clinical research protocols on average for four (4) hours per week...

*Administration/Service*: You will be expected to participate, to the extent that you may be reasonably called upon, in administrative and/or service functions of the Department and the Medical School...

Your salary for the 2004–2005 academic year will be at the annual rate of $_____. Thereafter, your compensation will be reviewed at least annually, and sources of funding and FTE allocations may change that may affect your salary.

The Department will cover the registration fee for the _____
board certification examination should you choose to take it. We encourage
you to do so. This reimbursement may be considered taxable income to you.

*Faculty Practice Plan; Clinical Services Agreement; Compliance with Medicare and
Medicaid Laws and Regulations; Mandatory Education*: You will become a mem-
ber of the _____ and be subject to its rules and the Faculty
Practice Plan. You will also be required to enter into a *Clinical Services Agree-
ment and Restrictive Covenant* with _____ and to comply with and
attend educational sessions on Medicare and Medicaid laws and regulations.
All patient care performed by you will be billed through the Faculty Practice
Plan, and the resulting income will be the property of _____.
A Faculty Practice Plan billing number will be issued to you prior to your
engaging in any patient care activities.

The _____ has adopted a *Code of Conduct*, a copy of
which is enclosed. As a condition of employment, you must acknowledge that
you have received, read and understood the *Code of Conduct*. The acknowledgement form is also enclosed and must be signed and returned.

*Additional Conditions of Appointment*. This offer of appointment is also subject
to the following:

1. Your agreement to comply with the bylaws, policies, and procedures of
   _____, including the *Information for Faculty* handbook, and the
   *Code of Conduct*;

2. Your obtaining and maintaining an unlimited _____ medical license
   and DEA registration;

3. Your acceptance by the _____ for professional
   liability (malpractice) insurance coverage;

4. Your obtaining and maintaining medical staff membership and clinical
   privileges at the hospital(s) where you will be assigned;

5. Your eligibility to participate in the Medicare and Medicaid programs,
   and your ability to be credentialed for treatment of managed care patients;
   and _____.

Your anticipated start date is dependent on the satisfaction of all conditions
specified in this letter. Because the process is time-sensitive, it is important
that you complete and return all required forms promptly. If you accept the
terms and conditions of the appointment contained in this letter of offer,
please sign and return one copy of the letter within the next two weeks, accompanied by the *Code of Conduct* acknowledgement form, Clinical Services

Agreement, Professional Liability Self-Insurance Questionnaire, and Credentialing Application completed according to the enclosed instructions.

Upon receipt of your signed acceptance of this offer and other required materials, and the satisfaction of all other conditions of appointment, we will forward our recommendations to our Dean's office for consideration.

Very truly yours,

Chair, Department of Psychiatry        Dean and Executive Vice President

Enclosures

ACCEPTANCE OF OFFER OF APPOINTMENT

I accept the offer of appointment described in this letter subject to all its terms and conditions.

_____
Signature

Print name: _____
Date: _____

# PART III

## Once You're There...

# CHAPTER 8

# Managing Your Time

Blythe A. Corbett, Ph.D.

Donald M. Hilty, M.D.

Your time is your life.

*Bryan Tracy*

A career in academic medicine is highly challenging, especially because of the recent emergence of the new category of faculty clinician-educator (Levinson et al. 1998). The strategies outlined in this chapter are designed to help you make the most of your most critical and limited resource: time. Among the factors that contribute to success for health educators is effective time management (Ransdell et al. 2001); the way we manage our time permits or inhibits every other activity outlined in this book, from manuscript preparation to mentorship to promotion.

Although the focus of this chapter is primarily on work activities, the ideas expressed are applicable to your personal life as well. In fact, by applying these simple tools, you will find more time to spend in the other important areas of your life; namely, family, friends, and leisure.

## TIME MANAGEMENT SKILLS AND THE FRONTAL LOBES

Those who make the worst use of their time are the first to complain of its brevity.

*Jean de la Bruyère*

There is recent evidence that the neural correlates of cognitive time management include several regions of the frontal lobe (dorsolateral prefrontal cortex, anterior cingulate gyrus, inferior prefrontal cortex) as well as supplemental motor areas. These areas have been found to be involved in various tasks of time estimation and motor timing (Rubia and Smith 2004). Furthermore, the frontal lobes are implicated in temporal processing or the sequencing of recent and remote events (McAndrews and Milner 1991; Milner et al. 1985; Moscovitch 1989; Shimamura et al. 1990). It is not surprising then that the aforementioned areas are also involved in executive functioning. Executive functions include self-regulatory skills that affect an individual's planning, flexibility, generation of information, inhibition of impulses, and problem-solving ability. Thus, we propose that effective time management requires intact and functional higher order or executive abilities—and perhaps requires skill development to ensure fitness.

## Executive Time Functions

Although the precise component processes of the executive functions are a matter of controversy, for the purpose of this chapter we have selected the following broadly defined executive domains that are directly or indirectly implicated in the ability to manage time effectively: attention, organization, inhibition, and parallel processing (defined below). We provide applications and guidelines to help you to better attend to, organize, manage, and respond to the challenges of managing your time effectively and efficiently.

- *Pay attention:* Attention is a broad and multifaceted term that includes the ability to attend (concentrate), direct our thought (focus), maintain focus (sustain), and shift our thought (switch).
- *Concentrate:* Concentration is needed to overcome the numerous visual, auditory, and social distractions in the academic work environment. The more you can do to control your environment and remove extraneous stimuli, the more able you will be to attend to the demands of your day. Suggestions include closing the office door, socializing outside of work, getting in to work early, focusing on challenging tasks in the morning when you are fresh, and creating an optimal work setting.
- *Focus:* Stick with a task until it is complete. Brian Tracy, the author of *Time Power* (2004), advises that you handle a piece of paper only once: either act on it, delegate it, file it, or discard it. In the process, you create a habit of being a master at task completion.

- *Sustain projects:* Create periods of time in which you know that you will not be interrupted. In your weekly schedule, build in blocks of time that will be used expressly for tasks that require sustained mental effort, such as grant writing and manuscript preparation. Protect this time religiously and do not be flexible with it (see *protected time* later in this chapter).
- *Switch flexibly:* The demands of academia require that you be mentally flexible and easily transition from one activity to the next. Prior to moving to the next activity, create a brief written or dictated note or memo to summarize any remaining activities so that you can easily pick up where you left off when you restart the activity. Ensuring that meetings end on time, and that there is a short break before the next one, will help with this task.

## Organization

At the heart of productivity are clear, organized, and systematic thoughts and actions. Success is an idea that has been acted on effectively, and highly effective people tend to be very organized. Many great ideas get lost or stolen because they are not acted on in an efficient or effective manner. Among the fundamental skills of good organization include creating ideas (generating), selecting the right goals (prioritizing), choosing the direction (planning), and acting on the ideas (implementing).

- *Generating:* Taking time to think is often the best use of your time. Allow yourself the chance to generate ideas and goals spontaneously and allow your mind to remain open and flexible. Get in the habit of promptly recording your ideas through dictation or in a notebook. Keep a file of new ideas and look at them and revise them at least once per month. Goal-setting theory predicts that specific and moderately difficult goals produce higher levels of performance than general, ambiguous, or easy goals (Locke 1968).
- *Prioritizing:* Emergency medical personnel are masters at prioritizing, a process referred to as triage. Similarly, successful people are masters at having clear, precise goals, which they routinely rewrite and review. Brian Tracy (2004) highlights that we have a natural tendency to work diligently on things that often need not be done at all. Thus, he recommends prioritizing your goals by assigning them with an *A* (essential to achieve), *B* (good to achieve), or *C* (nice to achieve) rating. In addition to your own needs, it is essentially important to

include the fundamental *A* goals of your academic department. Tracy further recommends that in the process of setting your priorities, you ask yourself "What is the consequence of not acting upon this goal?" Once you've assigned your ratings, transfer all your *A* goals to a separate piece of paper. Take action on your top goal by creating a detailed plan. In regard to other activities and requests that do not meet the *A* criteria, learn to say no.

- *Long-term planning:* Creating a plan for a long-term goal is like taking a trip, in that once you know your destination, you work backwards, planning the necessary route to get there. Break projects down into manageable, well-defined steps. In the process, draft a plan, create deadlines, and assign roles. One of the best-kept secrets of effective time management is delegating steps that can be assigned to other individuals. Make use of resources, systems, and personnel that are already accessible to you. Don't waste your precious time reinventing systems and templates that can facilitate goal achievement. However, with this said, if a system for doing something does not exist and will have future application, take the time to do it right the first time; create a foundation that is both endurable and flexible. For example, take the time to carefully draft and maintain a curriculum vitae, which you will need throughout your academic career, or report formats, which you will use frequently. In the process of planning your goals, keep in mind that as with all well-planned trips, there are always surprises, delays, and detours along the way. Highly successful people anticipate change, think ahead, plan for contingencies, and simultaneously create a plan B.
- *Short-term planning:* When you drive a car, you focus primarily on the area just ahead while you maintain a vague awareness of objects far in the distance and periphery. Similarly, you need to spend much of your energy targeted on goals in the immediate future; otherwise your short-term goals will ultimately all become long-term. Even so, your short-term goals should be thoughtfully and systematically linked to your long-term agenda. Ask yourself, "Is this objective or activity furthering me down the road, or is it a detour?"
- *Opportunistic organizing:* Every day situations arise that are not planned, such as meeting and appointment cancellations. Take full advantage of these opportunities and reinvest your time wisely. Resist the temptation to socialize or otherwise direct your energy in nonproductive ways.
- *Implementing:* Once you have dreamed big, selected a goal, and created a plan, take action. The most successful people invariably work from lists. The list you work from should consist of precise, systematic action

steps. Review your plan regularly and take action on your steps daily. Along the way, determine the critical steps that will prevent you from achieving your goal and work on that step first. Concentrate your energies initially on removing all factors that are self-limiting (e.g., training) or environment-limiting (e.g., funding, lab space) that are critical to achieving your overarching goal. Also, reward yourself for achieving your goals. Remember, reinforcement delivered immediately following a behavior increases the likelihood that the behavior will occur in the future (Thorndike 1911/1970). Managing work invariably includes prioritizing, organizing, completing, and balancing.

## Inhibition

Our brains, and the prefrontal cortex in particular, engage in an ongoing balance or neural interplay between inhibitory and excitatory activity (Knight and Stuss 2002). Similarly, our external world places numerous demands on our time, requiring a persistent balance between knowing when to act and when to inhibit our behavior. For example, it is very tempting to catch up on your e-mail between meetings, but one does not want to reply hastily, particularly on a sensitive issue; it is very easy to give bad news to others by e-mail rather than in person, but more time can be spent in the clean up than was saved. Although it takes emotional and behavioral control, a better plan is to sift through e-mails to see if there is one that needs immediate attention. Self-discipline is a critical personal attribute related to publication productivity among health educators (Ransdell et al. 2001). Yet productivity requires disciplining not only our behavior but our time. This means being punctual, starting and stopping meetings on time, delaying rewards, and structuring our schedule such that we have predetermined time to engage in our *A,* some *B,* and some *C* goals.

## Parallel Processing

The life of the academic research-educator is by definition multifaceted and requires the ability to identify, maintain, and act on many variables simultaneously. The more organized we are in approaching and managing our work life, the more systematic (system), efficient (speed of processing), effective (problem-solving), and productive (fluency) we can be.

- *System:* Highly productive people tend to be very systematic in their approach to their goals. Thus, it is important to establish routines and methods for executing tasks.

- *Speed of processing:* "Multitasking" is actually a misnomer: in truth, we can focus on only one priority at a time. Therefore, once a task is chosen, allow enough time to complete the job, maintain a steady pace, and complete it in excellent fashion (Tracy 2004). Find your working rhythm and stick with it; consistency in thought and action are hallmark features of great leaders. Work all the time you are at work—then go home.
- *Problem-solving:* Nearly everything we do presents us with a problem or conflict that requires a solution or action. The way we approach problems can often determine the consequences. The more cognitive control we have, the better we often are at generating good resolve. Tracy (2004) recommends the following: think before you act, write down the problem or crisis, delegate responsibility when someone else is more qualified, get the facts, and develop a policy on how to manage the situation in the future.
- *Fluency:* Productivity in our life goals involves organizational abilities that are associated with time, resource, computer, interpersonal, and self-management skills (Smith 1999). A useful technique is to visualize the process of goals being accomplished both internally and externally. Begin and plan your projects visually through the use of graphs, flowcharts, or storyboarding with index cards. The very act of writing and drafting out ideas on the computer helps to synthesize and solidify the achievement of them, but don't worry much about punctuation, phrasing, and other mechanics at this time.
- *Protected time:* Your time for career development needs to be estimated in advance of hire and protected, which means that it has to be negotiated in your contract. Once you have protected time, it should be used judiciously for critical activities that require extended periods of attention for completion, rather than for catching up on myriad day-to-day tasks.

## THE WHO, WHAT, WHEN, AND HOW OF TIME MANAGEMENT

> Our costliest expenditure is time.
>
> *Theophrastus*

It is essential that you answer for yourself the who, what, when, and how of time management. Set aside a few hours in the next week and write out related information based on your work situation.

- *Who:* Determine who is available to assist you in your career through mentorship, delegating responsibilities, and collaborating. These individuals may be supervisors, administrators, secretarial personnel, research assistants, students, networking groups, community resources, and volunteers.

- *What:* Determine your professional values and goals. If you have difficulty determining what these are, look at what you do, the materials that you read, and how you would like to spend your work time. Our goals are akin to a long-term research program; as we proceed through our academic inquiry, our questions and goals tend to get increasingly refined.
- *When:* Determine your priorities and set deadlines for goal achievement. Make sure to negotiate protected time as part of your contract. In contrast, also make sure to build in breaks (vacations) and rewards (reinforcement) along the way to celebrate your time well spent.
- *How:* Determine the ways in which you are going to accomplish your goals through planning and problem-solving strategies. The implementation of your plan should include the utilization of people, systems, technology, and other resources.

## SMART STRATEGIES

> The really efficient laborer will be found not to crowd his day with work, but will saunter to his task surrounded by a wide halo of ease and leisure.
>
> *Henry David Thoreau*

- *Use a planner:* You must have a planner and use it religiously. It doesn't matter if it is electronic (dictation, personal digital assistant [PDA]) or written, so long as it is accessible, efficient, and allows you to record daily, weekly, monthly, and yearly data.
- *List:* Always work from a list. Check off your items and transfer unfinished items to subsequent lists. Also, consider creating a sign to indicate tasks that you have completed but that depend on someone else for their final completion.
- *Use a filing system:* Establish an excellent filing system that includes an organizational strategy (e.g., alphabetical, chronological) that allows you to easily find your materials. Create time files based on both due dates and short-term and long-term goals. Take time to update your computer filing system every 6 months through editing, deletions, and additions.

- *Delegate:* Learn to delegate responsibilities to personnel whose job it is to complete given tasks. Also learn to delegate tasks to individuals who are more qualified during times of crisis. Spend more time training the staff who are working for you (this is a long-term investment).

- *Master your calendar:* Be the master of your calendar by setting your weekly schedule with research needs, departmental meetings, patient appointments, teaching assignments, and, of course, your personal time. Ensure that you have created larger blocks of time to focus on long-term projects that require sustained attention. At the end of each day, look ahead at the calendar for the next day.

- *Be consistent with your schedule:* Be punctual. Get a reputation for being somebody that people, especially you, can count on.

- *Prioritize meetings:* Avoid meetings that are not critical. So much time is wasted in unproductive, redundant, and politicized agendas. Run your meetings efficiently by providing a clear agenda, starting and stopping on time, and providing minutes to all attendees.

- *Organize your workspace:* When you prepare for a task, clear all other materials from your workspace and assemble all (and only) the necessary materials for the task at hand. This simple process helps to create an external sense of order for yourself—even if you feel an internal sense of chaos!

- *Manage the telephone:* There are a number of effective ways to manage the barrage of telephone interruptions, including having your calls screened, holding calls, setting clear callback times, batching calls, planning calls in advance, and taking good notes during conversations (Tracy 2004).

## QUESTIONS TO DISCUSS WITH A MENTOR OR COLLEAGUE

1. Who are the faculty and staff (resources) that can assist me with my position and goals?
2. What are the fundamental *A* goals of our academic department?
3. When and how much protected time can I obtain to pursue my academic goals?
4. How can I utilize the technology and department resources to facilitate the achievement of my academic, clinical, and research goals?
5. Will you review my short-term and long-term goals with me on a regular basis and provide me with feedback and guidance?

# REFERENCES

Knight RT, Stuss DT: Prefrontal cortex: the present and the future, in Principles of Frontal Lobe Functions. Edited by Stuss DT, Knight RT. New York, Oxford University Press, 2002, pp 573–597

Levinson W, Branch WT, Kroenke K: Clinician-educators in academic medical centers: a two-part challenge. Ann Intern Med 1:59–64, 1998

Locke EA: Toward a theory of task motivation and incentives. Organizational Behavior and Human Performance 3:157–189, 1968

McAndrews MP, Milner B: The frontal cortex and memory for temporal order. Neuropsychologia 29:849–859, 1991

Milner B, Petrides M, Smith ML: Frontal lobes and the temporal organization of memory. Hum Neurobiol 4:137–142, 1985

Moscovitch M: Confabulation and the frontal systems: strategic versus associative retrieval in neuropsychological theories of memory, in Varieties of Memory and Consciousness: Essays in Honour of Endel Tulving. Edited by Roediger HL 3rd, Craik FIM. Hillsdale, NJ, Lawrence Erlbaum, 1989, pp 133–160

Ransdell LB, Dinger MK, Cooke C, et al: Factors related to publication productivity in a sample of female health educators. Am J Health Behav 25:468–480, 2001

Rubia K, Smith A: The neural correlates of cognitive time management: a review. Acta Neurobiol Exp (Wars), 64:329–340, 2004

Shimamura AP, Janowsky JS, Squire LR: Memory for the temporal order of events in patients with frontal lobe lesions and amnesic patients. Neuropsychologia 28:803–813, 1990

Smith GR: Project leadership: why project management alone doesn't work. Hosp Mater Manage Q 21:88–92, 1999

Thorndike EL: Animal Intelligence. Darien, CT, Hafner, 1911/1970

Tracy B: Time Power. New York, AMACOM American Management Association, 2004

# ADDITIONAL RESOURCES

Applegate WB, Williams ME: Career development in academic medicine. Am J Med 89:263–267, 1990

Dartmouth University: Academic Skills Center [Web site]. Available at: http://www.dartmouth.edu/~acskills/success/time.html. Accessed March 3, 2005.

Mind Tools: Time management skills—maximize your effectiveness. Available at: http://www.mindtools.com/pages/main/newMN_HTE.htm. Accessed March 3, 2005.

Time Management Guide Team: Personal time management guide. Available at: http://www.time-management-guide.com/. Accessed March 3, 2005.

Verrier ED: Getting started in academic cardiothoracic surgery. J Thorac Cardiovasc Surg 119:4, S1–10, 2000

Zimmermann PG: Nursing secrets: managing our work life. Emerg Nurse 10:14–16, 2002

# CHAPTER 9

# Reading and Preparing a Basic Budget

David Peterson, M.B.A., FACMPE

Whether it is during a public policy debate over government planning, while managing personal investments and home decision-making, or in one's professional life, some type of budget or budget discussion will inevitably arise. This is especially true for the academic psychiatrist. Valuable management tools, budgets are commonly used in academic departments of psychiatry. The academic psychiatrist may be asked to read, draft, or comment on a budget in a variety of venues such as department planning, grant writing, clinical programming, or program development, to name a few. This chapter seeks to illustrate key elements of an academic budget, through examples and detailed definitions, and to present strategies for preparation, tracking, and maintenance of allocated funds.

## KEY CONCEPTS

In its simplest form, a budget is a forecast of revenues and expenses over a defined period of time (Dictionary.com 2005). *Revenues* can be derived from many different sources: grants, fees for professional services or the sale of products, or an allocation from a central institutional source. *Expenses* represent the cost of the resources necessary to generate the revenues and can include things such as personnel, fringe benefits, supplies, equipment, travel, and rent. *Budgets* are usually expressed in periods of a year, often defined as a *fiscal year*, although budgets can be developed for any period of time. Fiscal years and calendar years can coincide; however, fiscal years are usually defined by the business cycle of the organization (Philanthropic

Research Inc. 2005). For academic institutions, the fiscal year is frequently tied to the academic year or defined as a period beginning on July 1 and ending on June 30 of the following year. The academic psychiatrist will likely also encounter a *grant year*, which is a function of the funding cycle followed by the granting agency. For most extramurally funded grants, the grant year can begin and end anytime during the calendar year and can certainly straddle an institution's fiscal years.

The goal of a budget is to closely match revenues and expenses to determine a level of *profitability* (expressed as a positive number) or *loss* (expressed as a negative number or set off by parentheses) and to determine the level of resources (expenses) a program or activity will require to be successful. Budgets contain forecasts of future activity and are based on a series of assumptions. Although they may appear *static*, a good budget will be *dynamic* and have the capability to respond to a changing environment.

The *matching* of revenues and expenses is a principal accounting concept and is a critical element when developing a budget that is intended to portray as accurately as possible the revenues and expenses attached to a program or activity in a defined period. The more accurate of two accounting methods for matching revenues and expenses is the *accrual basis method*, a method that recognizes a revenue or expense when it occurs, regardless of when the actual cash for the transaction is collected or expended. The other accepted method for accounting for revenues and expenses is the *cash basis method*, which recognizes a revenue and expense transaction in the period when cash is exchanged, not when the activity occurred (Welsch et al. 1979).

For the health care field and clinical group practices—an increasingly important component of an academic department—the principal method of accounting for revenues and expenses is the cash (or modified cash) basis (Ross et al. 1991). As a result, academic budgets usually reflect when cash is expected to be collected or expended.

## WORKING WITH BUDGETS

A budget is not a plan in itself but is one of several documents in support of an overall business plan and strategy (Kotler 1980). To be useful, a budget needs to be monitored throughout the fiscal year so that actual performance can be measured against the budgeted forecast. *Actual versus budget* comparisons can be made as frequently as necessary, but they are most often made monthly, quarterly, semi-annually, and certainly annually, depending on the business cycle, seasonality, or activity that is to be measured. Deviations from the budget and the difference between actual results and the budgeted forecast are *variances* (Horngren et al. 2002). Variances are conventionally expressed as percentage differences and can be expressed in either positive or negative terms.

## A Basic Budget

A proposed budget describes a projection of revenue and associated expenses for a defined period of time. Figure 9–1 is an example of a generally accepted format for a proposed annual budget.

Budgets can provide much more detail than what is shown in Figure 9–1. For example, the category "Personnel" often lists specific individuals or positions that devote effort to the program. In this example, more detail may also be required in listing the individual components that make up "Supplies," "Travel," and "Equipment." Even more detail is usually supplied in a *budget narrative,* which describes the underlying assumptions used to develop the budget. The narrative describes how the revenues were derived and why the expenses are necessary.

## TRACKING INFORMATION OVER TIME

Once the budget is developed and approved, it becomes a useful gauge of the progress of a program or activity throughout the period being evaluated. Figure 9–2 illustrates a monthly comparison of the $120,000 in revenues (budgeted in Figure 9–1) compared with the actual revenues that were realized.

When evaluating the actual revenue performance against the budgeted performance in Figure 9–2, it becomes evident that the program or activity was slightly ahead of budget ($50,433 actual vs. $50,000 budgeted) in November but began to slip behind the totals budgeted in December ($59,189 actual vs. $60,000 budgeted). Moreover, the program or activity director can see that although this slip became more pronounced in the subsequent months, actual revenues began to recover toward the end of the period. This becomes clearer when the data in Figure 9–2 are displayed in a *line graph* (Figure 9–3).

Tracking of variances and comparison of actual versus budgeted performance over time can be represented nicely through line graphs. In this instance, time increments are usually represented on the $x$ axis and dollars (or units) are usually represented on the $y$ axis. Using the data provided in Figure 9–2, Figure 9–3 illustrates a typical line graph, comparing actual revenues against the budgeted revenues projected in Figure 9–1 over a 12-month period.

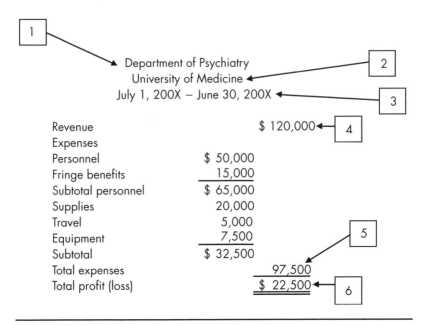

**FIGURE 9–1.**   Example of proposed annual budget.

The key elements of this proposed budget describe 1) the program or activity it represents, 2) the organization the program or activity is a part of, 3) the period of time the budget represents, 4) estimated revenues, 5) the expenses necessary to support these revenues, and 6) the difference between the revenues and expenses as either a profit or loss (double underlined).

The graph in Figure 9–3 shows that the "Cumulative actual" line and the "Budget" line begin to vary significantly from each other in February but trend toward merging again in May and June. From this graph, it is visually evident that the actual revenue collected began to drop off in the last 6 months of the year. Identifying this *trend* allows the program director or activity director to make adjustments in expenses where appropriate.

## KEY CONCEPTS AND DEFINITIONS

**Accrual basis accounting:** A method of accounting that records when a revenue or expense occurs, rather than when the revenue or expense was actually collected or expended.

**Budget:** A forecast of revenues and expenses over a defined period of time.

**Budget narrative:** A written summary that describes the assumptions and details contained in a budget document.

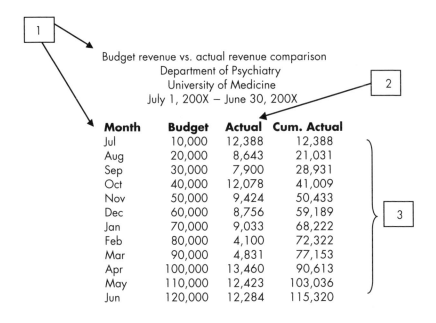

FIGURE 9–2. Monthly comparison of budgeted and realized revenues.

The figure shows 1) a descriptive header and column identifiers, 2) actual revenue activity by month, and 3) a "cumulative actual" column that allows a comparison over a period of time of actual revenues against those that were budgeted.

**Cash basis accounting:** A method of accounting that records a revenue or expense when it is actually collected or expended.

**Fiscal year:** A 12-month period that may coincide with the calendar year but is most often defined by the business cycle of the organization.

**Line graph:** A type of graph that is useful in tracking actual revenues and expenses to budgeted revenues and expenses over a period of time.

**Matching:** An accounting principle that describes the pairing of revenues and expenses to an activity or event.

**Variance:** A measurement of a deviation between budgeted or forecasted performance and actual performance. Variances can be either positive or negative.

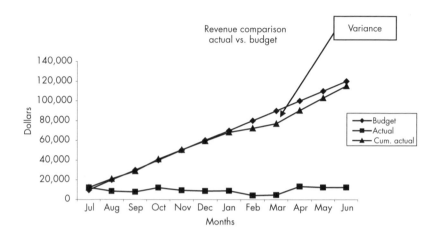

**FIGURE 9–3.**    Cumulative actual variance.

## SMART STRATEGIES

Whether the academic psychiatrist is drafting or evaluating a budget, some smart budget strategies include the following:

- *Test the assumptions behind the budget:* Are all of the expenses and revenues associated with the activity represented? Are the expenses reasonable and defensible? Are the assumptions realistic?
- *Check if the budget is complete:* Is there a descriptive title? Is the period identified? Do the numbers add up?
- *Evaluate the percentage change in revenues and expenses:* When comparing like budgets from period to period, review the percentage change in revenues and expenses. Are expenses growing faster than revenues? Are revenues and expenses matched to the appropriate period?
- *Identify the overall trend:* Are revenues and expenses growing or declining appropriately? In an annual budget, 1 month of actual data does not make a trend. It usually takes several months of actual data to identify a trend. Line graphs, as illustrated in Figure 9–3, are a useful tool in identifying trends.
- *Read the notes or narrative accompanying the budget:* The notes and narrative will often describe critical budget assumptions and help the reader evaluate whether realistic or unrealistic budget assumptions have been made.

In summary, a budget is one component of a business plan that matches revenues and expenses over a defined period of time. It describes the resources necessary to complete the activity or support the program as well as any revenues that will arise from that activity or program. Finally, once developed, budgets can be used throughout the year to track actual performance to that which was budgeted and be one measure of a program or activity's success or failure.

## QUESTIONS TO DISCUSS WITH A MENTOR OR COLLEAGUE

1. What activities in a department of psychiatry can be budgeted and how can they be measured and tracked?
2. When will revenues and expenses for a program or activity exactly match?
3. What would be a reasonable percentage increase to inflate salaries and benefits annually, and what are the implications if there is no increase?
4. When might there be no revenues attached to a program or activity and only expenses?

## REFERENCES

Dictionary.com: [Lexico Publishing Group, LLC Web site]. Available at: http://dictionary.reference.com. Accessed February 11, 2005.

Horngren CT, Sunden GL, Stratton WO: Introduction to Management Accounting, 13th Edition. Upper Saddle River, NJ, Prentice-Hall, 2002

Kotler P: Marketing Management, 4th Edition. Upper Saddle River, NJ, Prentice-Hall, 1980

Philanthropic Research, Inc.: Glossary [Guidestar Web site]. Available at: http://www.guidestar.org/help/glossary.jsp. Accessed February 11, 2005.

Ross A, Williams S, Schafer E: Ambulatory Care Management, 2nd Edition. Albany, NY, Delmar , 1991

Welsch G, Zlatkovich C, Harrison W, et al: Intermediate Accounting, 5th Edition. Homewood, IL, Irwin, 1979

# Aligning Your Goals With Those of Colleagues, the Department, and the Institution

Donald M. Hilty, M.D.

Robert E. Hales, M.D., M.B.A.

In order to be successful, faculty members must balance their individual goals with those of the department and the school of medicine. When recruited to an institution, a faculty member often receives a formal letter that summarizes the department's commitment along with other issues discussed during the interview process (see Chapters 6 and 7 of this volume). However, not everything can be fully documented, and ongoing negotiation of individual and institutional interests are necessary. As the career of a faculty member progresses, it is common for him or her to make a shift in interests and goals. Therefore, facilitating communication, building common goals, and developing flexibility on the part of both the faculty member and the institution are important ingredients for success. In addition, a process that monitors the achievement of personal and institutional goals should be in place to provide constructive feedback to the individual faculty member and the department.

In today's challenging managed care environment, faculty and academic departments in American medical schools are under considerable pressure not only to publish but to generate revenue from clinical activities to support their educational and research missions (Longnecker et al. 2003). Publications demonstrate how clinical departments in a variety of disciplines have succeeded in generating adequate revenue to support their teaching and research missions (Brandt et al. 2002; Guss 2002; Schindler et al. 2002; Shea et al. 1996). This chapter will review common denominators of these plans, which increase faculty clinical productivity, enhance research and scholarly activity, and improve overall career satisfaction (Hales et al., in press).

## INITIAL AND ONGOING ALIGNMENT

There are five general areas that categorize the many university and academic activities that faculty members engage in: clinical work, research, teaching, administration, and community service. Faculty interests vary over time and according to academic rank and academic series. For example, a faculty member who is in a clinician-educator academic series may choose to focus on clinical care and teaching, whereas someone focused on a research career would choose differently. Coming to an agreement on these choices between the faculty member and department early on is part of the negotiation described in Chapter 12 of this book. Regardless of faculty preferences, an annual fiscal review can evaluate financial viability for all parties.

It is important for a faculty member to assess how his or her goals align with the goals of others at the institution before hiring, during the early stages of the appointment, and periodically during the time spent at that institution (e.g., every 4–8 years). For example, most clinician-educators deliver clinical care, teach, administer a program, and provide community service. A faculty member may consider the following questions to determine what is possible and feasible. The following are examples of questions one could ask oneself to determine what goals are feasible:

*Do my individual academic goals align with department and institutional goals?*
- Should I develop a center on technology if it is not highly valued? (No.)
- Should I develop a center on women's mental health? (Yes, one is needed nearly everywhere.)

*Do others share my interests and want to collaborate?*
- Should I start basic science research in a proven program when there are two others to collaborate with and an on-site mentor? (Yes.)
- Should I start educational research in the absence of two or three

other educational researchers in the department or school? (Maybe not, unless you can wholly support the infrastructure and have sufficient drive.)

*Are there resources (time, funds, other) for such research ?*
- Will there be sufficient time to evaluate educational initiatives without protected time or with a heavy teaching load? (No.)
- Is seed money or other funds available to start pilot projects, in order to get to a larger grant? (If yes, start planning.)

One of the most difficult aspects of this process is that faculty members may not be completely sure what they want to do. In that case, early career faculty may try a mix of activities to clarify interests and thereby help the department meet its needs as well as its service obligations to the community. This works well as long as there is an understanding that priorities may change over time for both the faculty member and the department.

## CHANGE

The academic environment is prone to significant change, particularly in the current economic climate. Change may work for or against the achievement of individual and departmental goals. A decrease in income (e.g., contracts, grants) may necessitate a change in plans. Likewise, individual and other faculty goals may change (e.g., key collaborators may leave, personal or family issues may arise). Change of a division head or department chair is also a significant event, because the direction of the department may shift. Similar to the investment world (in which one needs a diversified portfolio), in academic life it is helpful to have a marketable area (or two) of expertise that is adaptable to various changes. Another key to versatility is building relationships with many individuals and not excluding anyone.

## MEETING RESPONSIBILITIES AND EARNING FAIR CREDIT

Usually, department chairs and faculty have a general sense as to whether individuals have met their occupational responsibilities and whether they have been given due credit for a particular duty. The hallmark of this is a good working relationship, flexibility for the betterment of the team, and the success of all parties. Sometimes, responsibility and credit are hard to assess, particularly in large departments. Other times, faculty are involved with more things than the department chair is aware of or ordinary tasks and positions become complicated. In these situations, an operational evaluation of responsibility and credit may be in order.

To highlight one institution's reward system for educational and research productivity, the Department of Psychiatry and Behavioral Sciences at the University of California (UC), Davis, developed a faculty practice plan in 1998 that assigned a monetary value to various educational and research activities that occurred that year. Faculty members have three components to their salary: a base, a differential, and a bonus. The *base* is derived from the UC salary schedule according to rank (assistant, associate, or full professor) and step within the rank and is given to support educational and research missions. The *differential* (see Appendices 10–A, B, and C) is negotiated annually with the department chair and is tied to generating clinical revenue or to participation in additional research and departmental or school educational activities. The *bonus* is paid when a faculty member has earned clinical income or has generated educational or research credit beyond what is required to cover his or her salary (over 100%).

In their annual meetings with the department chair, UC Davis faculty members are assigned a *salary goal,* which is the amount of money or academic credits necessary to cover 1) their salary, 2) fringe benefits, and 3) a departmental academic assessment (overhead, other) that is charged against total compensation and fringe benefits. The system is also a way to register faculty activities and give due credit, particularly to teaching—an issue that affects the livelihood of clinicians, clinical scholars, and researchers. An incentive system was developed for many responsibilities:

- Teaching and academic responsibilities (Table 10–1)
- Administrative and clinical activities: percentage of effort credits against their total compensation and benefits for selected departmental teaching and academic responsibilities (Appendix A)
- Scholarship and community service: credit is given as a percentage of their base salary and is based on the faculty member's activities for the previous year (Appendix B)
- Research grants: percentage of base salary, with consideration for 1) whether the granting agency is federal or nonfederal and 2) the annual direct costs of the grant (Appendix C).

The effective date of the first year of this compensation plan was July 1, 1999. The number of faculty increased 11.4% between July 1, 1999, and June 30, 2003, from 35 to 39 faculty members. Increases oc-

**TABLE 10–1.**    Departmental teaching and academic responsibilities[a]

| Activity | Credit |
| --- | --- |
| Co-director, Doctoring I, II, or III (a 26-week, half-day course for first, second, and third year medical students) | 10% |
| Director, Psychiatry 403 (second-year psychiatry course) | 20% |
| Director of Faculty Development | 10% |
| Chair, Diversity Advisory Committee | 10% |
| Chair, Psychiatry Academic Council | 10% |
| Chair, Ground Rounds Committee | 10% |
| Individual resident supervision (1 hour/week minimum) | 2% |
| Faculty mentoring | 1% |
| Department-based teaching[b] | 100% of contact hours |
| University-based teaching[b] | 50% of contact hours |

[a]Lectures, small group facilitator, lab instructor, case conference consultant, applicant interviews, and faculty development teaching.
[b]Credit for these activities is given as a percentage of base salary ($x$).

curred in the total dollar value of grants per faculty member (276.8%), total number of peer-reviewed papers (46.3%), and total number of publications (21.6%; both peer reviewed and non–peer reviewed, such as book chapters or books) (Appendix D).

## ADMINISTRATION: ESTABLISHING MUTUAL GOALS

Certain steps on the parts of both the faculty member and the department can facilitate setting joint goals, monitoring progress, and making adjustments (Table 10–2). An annual meeting with the department chair can help parties decide what research and activities to continue, discontinue, and begin—with all parties' interests maintained, with some compromises. This should occur early in the year, in February or March, in case plans need to be made, rather than at the end of the academic year in June. An annual report of academic activities (a computation of scholarly and research accomplishments) may be collected from the entire faculty prior to their meetings with the department chair. Finally, meetings and consultations with others may be necessary for resolving ongoing obstacles or making key career decisions.

**TABLE 10–2.**   Faculty and administration guidelines for success in maintaining joint goals

| Activity | Description/logistics | Faculty preparation | Administrative preparation |
|---|---|---|---|
| Annual meeting of each faculty member with administration | To be held early enough in the year (e.g., in February) to plan for next year | Prepare three objectives, a one-page CV, plans for next year, and a list of activities to discontinue | Assess department needs, issues, assessment of "let-go" items, and vision |
| Annual report from each faculty member | Includes publications, grants, and presentations; a "snapshot" of productivity | Two-page document | Template to use and prompt to do |
| Meetings as needed | Opportunities for individual and/or department that may require change urgently, if exercised | Half-page description of opportunity and options for change | Assessment of feasibility for individual and department |
| Consult | Obtain technical input/advice from faculty at other institutions | Identify problem, obstacle, decision, and/or question | Obtain input from trusted faculty |

## CONCLUSIONS

If incentives for faculty effort are aligned fairly and objectively, whether they are for research, scholarly, or clinical activities, the results should be robust and gratifying for the faculty member, the department chair, and the department. The allocation of a dollar value to specific educational and research activities provides tangible, financial incentives to faculty so they will devote both time and energy to this work. However, a financial incentive plan must be objective and fair to be successful (Brandt et al. 2002). Financial incentives for education and research may also be used with other successful interventions, including advanced degrees or fellowships (Ferrer and Katerndahl 2002), a faculty development curriculum (Neale et al. 2003), and unrestricted research grants for young faculty (Mavis and Katz 2003).

## SMART STRATEGIES

- Once per year, write out your top three goals and link those with departmental goals.
- Meet with your chair once per year to discuss goals, new plans, and options for trimming old initiatives.
- Help out the department chair by being a team player if asked to do something over the next year.
- Prepare a one- to two-page summary of key accomplishments for the year to go over with your department chair, so he or she knows some of the things you have done.
- Collaborate with others to build teamwork, increase productivity, and earn your salary, benefits, and incentives.

## QUESTIONS TO DISCUSS WITH A MENTOR OR COLLEAGUE

1. In what ways do my goals align or not align with the department's goals?
2. Is my department chair (and any other supervisor) aware of all that I am doing?
3. If I do not feel positive about one of the things I have to do, could I do something else to serve the department (and enjoy it) and is there someone else to whom I could give this activity (who might enjoy it)?
4. Am I being a team player, overall, to my trainees, colleagues, chair, department, and institution?
5. Do I have a diversified portfolio of interests to adapt to change if it occurs in the institution and if I want to stay put?

## REFERENCES

Brandt TL, Romme CR, LaRusso NF, et al: A novel incentive system for faculty in an academic medical center. Ann Intern Med 137:738–743, 2002

Ferrer RL, Katerndahl DA: Predictors of short-term and long-term scholarly activity by academic faculty: a departmental case study. Fam Med 34:455–461, 2002

Guss DA: A simple plan—faculty compensation in an academic department of emergency medicine. Acad Emerg Med 9:619–620, 2002

Hales RE, Shahrokh NC, Servis ME: A faculty practice plan designed to reward educational and research productivity. Acad Psychiatry (in press)

Longnecker DE, Henson DE, Wilczek K, et al: Future directions for academic practice plans: thoughts on organization and management from Johns Hopkins University and the University of Pennsylvania. Acad Med 78:1130–1143, 2003

Mavis B, Katz M: Evaluation of a program supporting scholarly productivity for new investigators. Acad Med 78:757–765, 2003

Neale AV, Schwartz KL, Schenk MJ, et al: Scholarly development of clinician faculty using evidence-based medicine as an organizing theme. Med Teach 25:442–447, 2003

Schindler N, Winchester DP, Sherman H: Recognizing clinical faculty's contributions in education. Acad Med 77:940–941, 2002

Shea S, Nickerson KG, Tenenbaum J, et al: Compensation to a department of medicine and its faculty members for the teaching of medical students and house staff. N Engl J Med 334:162–167, 1996

# APPENDIX 10–A
## DEPARTMENTAL ADMINISTRATIVE RESPONSIBILITIES[a]

| Activity | Credit |
|---|---|
| Department chair | 50% |
| Vice chair for Education | 20% |
| Vice chair for Research | 20% |
| Director, Forensic Psychiatry Division | 20% |
| Director, Child and Adolescent Psychiatry Division | 20% |
| Director, Consultation-Liaison Psychiatry Service | 20% |
| Medical Director, Psychiatry Outpatient Service | 20% |
| Director, Adult Psychiatry Residency Program | 40% |
| Director, Child Psychiatry Residency Program | 20% |
| Director, Forensic Psychiatry Training Program | 10% |
| Director, Psychology Training Program | 10% |
| Director, Medical Student Clerkship | 30% |
| Consultation psychiatry service coverage | 20% per day |

[a] Credit for these activities is given as a percentage of total compensation and benefits (e.g., if a faculty member's total compensation and benefits amount to $100,000, service as director of the medical student clerkship counts as 30%, or $30,000).

# APPENDIX 10–B
# SCHOLARSHIP AND COMMUNITY SERVICE[a]

| Publications | Credit |
|---|---|
| Primary author—peer reviewed | 5% |
| Co-author—peer reviewed | 4% |
| Primary author—non-peer reviewed | 3% |
| Co-author—non-peer reviewed | 2% |
| Book editor or co-editor | 10% |
| Book author or co-author | 10% |
| **Community service** | |
| Professional society officer or board member of national organization | 2% |
| Member study section | 5% |
| Member, ad hoc or special emphasis panel | 2% |
| Editor—peer-reviewed journal | 5% |
| Editorial board—peer-reviewed journal | 2% |
| Editorial board—non-peer-reviewed publication | 1% |
| Chair or co-chair, school of medicine, medical center, health system, or university committee | 3% |
| Member, school of medicine, medical center, health system, or university committee | 2% |
| Faculty sponsor or mentor, National Institutes of Health (NIH) career development award (K award or equivalent) | 5% |

[a]Credit for these activities is given as a percentage of base salary ($x$). It is based on the faculty member's activities for the previous year and must be documented at the time of the meeting with the department chair. Credit will not be given for in-press publications.

# APPENDIX 10-C
## ANNUAL DIRECT COSTS FROM GRANTS[a]

| <u>Type of grant</u> | <u>Credit</u>[a] |
|---|---|
| Nonfederal $1,000–$10,000 | 3% |
| Nonfederal $10,001–$50,000 | 5% |
| Nonfederal over $50,000 | 10% |
| Federal (NIH, National Institute of Mental Health, etc.) $1,000–$50,000 annual direct costs | 10% |
| Federal $50,001–$200,000 annual direct costs | 15% |
| Federal over $200,000 annual direct costs | 20% |

[a] Credit for annual direct costs charged to grants is given as a percentage of base salary ($x$).

## APPENDIX 10–D

## GRANTS AND PUBLICATIONS AT INITIATION OF SALARY PLAN AND AFTER 4 YEARS

| Grants | As of June 30, 1999 | As of June 30, 2003 |
|---|---|---|
| Number of grants | 25 | 61 |
| Total dollar value of all grants | $9,258,932 | $38,850,756 |
| Total number of faculty | 35 | 39 |
| Grants per faculty member | 0.71 | 1.56 |
| Total value of grants per faculty member | $264,541 | $996,173 |
| **Publications** | | |
| Total number of peer-reviewed publications | 67 | 98 |
| Total number of other publications | 35 | 26 |
| Total number of all publications | 102 | 124 |
| Total number of faculty | 35 | 39 |
| Peer-reviewed publications per faculty member | 1.91 | 2.51 |
| All publications per faculty member | 2.91 | 3.17 |

# Understanding and Preparing for the Process of Academic Promotion

Dan-Vy Mui, M.D.

Donald M. Hilty, M.D.

James A. Clardy, M.D.

Understanding the promotion and tenure (PandT) process at your institution is essential to your academic success. As you embark on your career, the PandT policies provide guidelines so you can set professional goals and map out how to accomplish them. By charting your course, you ensure that your hard work is actually propelling you in the desired direction. Along the way, you will compile an academic portfolio, a purposeful collection of materials that give evidence of what you have done. The most successful portfolios are the result of careful planning, not just a scrapbook of random endeavors. That is, you want to plan your journey toward promotion in such a way as to get good souvenirs.

It is important to realize that the key concepts and suggestions presented here are generalized. Be aware that different institutions may have different expectations. For this reason, you will want to access your institution's own PandT documents and ask questions of a mentor in your department who is well versed in the process.

## KEY CONCEPTS AND DEFINITIONS

Promotion and tenure often go together but are actually distinct processes and, on occasion, become disassociated from each other. *Promotion* is the process of ascending academic ranks based on established criteria. The levels to which you may be assigned begin with instructor and progress through assistant professor, associate professor, and finally professor. To be promoted, you must demonstrate that you are developing experience and expertise, that you have been productive, and that you have earned professional recognition. Promotion is recommended by your department and is approved by the institution's PandT committee and, ultimately, by the dean.

The *instructor* level is generally appropriate for those with limited experience. With the backing of your department chair and perhaps formal presentation in front of a PandT committee, you advance to the next level, attaining the status of assistant professor. The trigger for promotion may be obtaining board certification or some other milestone.

At institutions where there are defined time parameters for advancement, your tenure track "clock" will typically start at the *assistant professor* level. It is at this stage that you are really expected to demonstrate your potential. Often, you are given a time frame of 6–7 years to advance to the associate professor level.

To become an *associate professor,* you need to have proven capabilities in your field and are usually expected to assume more of a leadership and mentorship role. At some institutions, there remains a time frame for expected advancement. However, at many schools, there is no time frame at this stage and faculty may choose to remain at this level without being promoted to professor.

*Professor* status probably has the most variable criteria from institution to institution. In general, you need to have evidence of national or international prominence and leadership. This may be judged in the form of grants, publications, service in national and international organizations, and distinct contributions to the field.

With promotion usually comes progression along a *tenure* track, but some faculty choose not to seek tenure. Tenure at a medical school is different from that status in other academic settings and is difficult to define because its implications vary depending on the school. Once you have achieved tenure, it is associated with some security in position. You have proved that you are accomplished and may gain the right to more academic freedom. Perhaps even more important is the *process* of working toward tenure. Faculty who are attempting to gain tenure are more often given opportunities for academic nurturing and leadership.

Usually, you apply for tenure at the same time you apply for promotion from assistant to associate professor. If tenure is denied, this will be detrimental to your standing: you may be asked to leave, or you may have to assume responsibilities that are not in line with your goals if you remain at the institution.

Schools have different *tracks* or pathways through which you may earn promotion and tenure. The tracks differ in their emphasis on the various components of an academic position: research, teaching, clinical, and administrative duties. It is crucial to know which tracks are available at your institution because the names for tracks may carry significantly different connotations at different schools. Clinical attending or research scientist pathways are often highly regarded but are designated as nontenure tracks. A typical track is illustrated in Table 11–1.

## UNDERSTANDING CRITERIA FOR PROMOTION

Again, it is important to take the time to read the PandT guidelines at your institution, making sure that you are on the right track. Remember that the PandT expectations reflect what your job is *supposed* to be. Analyze the actual time you spend in various activities in a typical week or month. Negotiate with your department chair or his or her designee to better align your duties with your track. You want to consider 1) your goals, 2) what the department chair needs, 3) what the department needs, and 4) what the institution needs. It is important to be of service to your institution, not just your department (see Chapter 10).

If you are still in doubt about your own goals, it is better to wait to get on the tenure "clock" if possible. Use the time to explore possibilities, make relationships, start research, and be productive. Even when you are on the clock, you can take some time to try different avenues for the first 1–2 years. As your goals come into focus and your career evolves, you should continue reevaluating and renegotiating to stay in alignment with your pathway. You might take on new things, or you might dispense with others that make your path look like it has no direction—like Brownian movement. For example, if your reputation for excellent teaching earns you awards and an offer to be a clerkship director, it would enhance your development in a clinician educator track. Conversely, if you were instead assigned a large teaching duty while in a clinician scientist track, you would need to seriously consider how such an activity would affect your research productivity (most likely, the job should be declined). Many institutions have a mechanism for

**TABLE 11–1.**   Example components of typical track

|  | Tenure tracks | | | Nontenure tracks | |
| --- | --- | --- | --- | --- | --- |
|  | Basic scientist | Clinical scientist | Clinical educator | Research scientist | Clinical attending |
| Teaching | 10%–35% | 10%–50% | 10%–65% | 0%–10% | 0%–10% |
| Research | 50%–85% | 15%–85% | 5%–15% | 90%–100% | 0%–10% |
| Service (clinical, administrative) | 5%–35% | 5%–75% | 30%–85% | 0% | 80%–100% |

switching tracks before you come up for PandT consideration, but you will only be able to do this on a limited basis and should do so with caution.

You must be able to show evidence of what you are doing. Therefore, be mindful of documentation requirements at the onset—it is much easier to keep track of these things as you go along (see Chapter 5). Thinking about your work as a product and about how that product might later be packaged will help you in compiling your portfolio. In research, your products are your publications and presentations. Educational endeavors are sometimes more of a challenge to document. Always ask for evaluations when you teach, and be assertive about getting others to complete peer teaching evaluations.

## PREPARING AN ACADEMIC PORTFOLIO

You will be compiling a portfolio of your academic activity; the contents can include papers, books and chapters, evaluations, curricula, and educational material such as CD-ROMs or videos (see Chapter 4). Most institutions also give you the option of writing a short letter as well to accompany the contents of your portfolio. If your school does not provide a prototype of a portfolio and letter, ask your colleagues who have successfully attained promotion and tenure whether they would be willing to show you theirs as models.

Use your portfolio to highlight components of your curriculum vitae and activities that are most pertinent to your track. Instead of merely listing your accomplishments, consider how you want to package them to show a progression. For instance, demonstrate that your publications were cited by others and led to invited presentations. Rather than just stating that you started a new lecture series, describe how you used pre- and posttests to demonstrate effectiveness and then wrote it up in a paper.

The department chair will likely request letters of recommendation (see Chapter 18), and your institution may have guidelines as to how much you can facilitate that process. If it is allowed at your institution, you might ask in advance whether a contact feels comfortable writing you a letter. It is helpful for letters to come from highly regarded sources who are able to comment on your various qualifications. One source may be better able to discuss your clinical abilities; another may focus on your teaching skills. Your department chair or his or her representative will also contribute a letter. To make it easier for persons writing a recommendation, they should be provided with copies of your curriculum vitae that have the most relevant parts highlighted as well as a copy of your school's PandT requirements, again with the most relevant parts highlighted.

Do not let portfolio deficiencies detract from your work. Watch for these common, avoidable errors:

- Lack of documentation
- Activities that do not reflect reported time distributions
- Inadequate (or absent) evaluations of teaching
- Outside letter of recommendation not sufficient or appropriate
- Inappropriate track designation

## CONCLUSIONS

It is important to know the specific promotion and tenure process at your institution. Once you are aware of the requirements, keep them in mind as you map out your job to fit the tenure track. Continually evaluate your duties to make sure that you stay on target with your goals, and don't divert too many of your resources to going off on tangents. Think ahead about how to package your accomplishments to show evidence of your development, and avoid the common portfolio pitfalls. Being mindful of your destination at the onset will help ensure that you reach your goals.

## SMART STRATEGIES

- Reflect with your mentor on which opportunities to take or not take.
- Discuss with your mentor how your individual professional development can contribute to the success of the department.
- Meet collaborators outside of your department.
- Establish a network of peers and mentors outside of your institution.
- Attend national meetings and ask successful role models for their ideas and for possible collaborations.

## QUESTIONS TO DISCUSS WITH A MENTOR OR COLLEAGUE

1. How are tenure tracks defined at this institution?
2. What does my department value?
3. Who has been successful in doing what I want to do, and how did they do it?
4. Are examples of successful tenure packets available?
5. What opportunities (departmental jobs) are available that would benefit both my own career and the department or institution?

# ADDITIONAL RESOURCES

Academic Medicine [Academic Medicine Web site]. Available at: http://www .academicmedicine.org. Accessed March 7, 2005.

Association for Academic Psychiatry [Association for Academic Psychiatry Web site]. Available at: www.academicpsychiatry.org. Accessed March 7, 2005.

Glick TH: How best to evaluate clinician-educators and teachers for promotion? Acad Med 77:392–397, 2002

Lemkau JP, Ahmed SM: Helping junior faculty become published scholars. Acad Med 74:1264–1267, 1999

McHugh PR: A "letter of experience" about faculty promotion in medical schools. Acad Med 69:877–881, 1994

National Library of Medicine [PubMed Web site; search "faculty mentoring"]. Available at: www.pubmed.com. Accessed March 7, 2005.

# CHAPTER 12

# Negotiating With the Department Chair

## Jerald Belitz, Ph.D.

Academic life begins. The contract is signed, clinical and teaching assignments have commenced, and research projects are being conceptualized. It is now time to initiate the process of navigating the multiple demands and politics of the department and negotiating with the department chair for one's specific goals. Proficiency as a negotiator is critical for a meaningful and purposeful career. The requisite skills include the identification of personal values and passions, recognition of the assumptions and values of the department chair and other faculty, appreciation of the importance of finances, and engagement in creative problem solving.

## PERSONAL VALUES

### Mission

New faculty members have several important decisions to craft during the first 3 years of their careers: designating a promotion and tenure track, selecting research interests, and determining clinical populations with which to specialize. However, the most salient task is the definition of a personal mission and purpose (Citrin and Smith 2003; Cohen 2003; Russo and Schoemaker 2002; Seaman 1999).

Professional satisfaction results from determining one's passion and strengths and creating a vision that focuses on accomplishments that are larger than the individual. Missions that are inherently self-serving are precluded, such as becoming the youngest department chair in the history of academic psychiatry. Visions that provide purpose can be relatively limited, such as developing evidence-based treatment protocols for patients with traumatic brain injury and co-occurring psychiatric diagnoses; or more generalized, such as constructing a comprehensive system of care that provides mental health care to underserved populations. Every endeavor can and should advance the realization of this vision.

Decisions regarding professional objectives need to be calibrated with a clear vision of one's personal life. Brown and colleagues (2003) analyzed data collected from four groups of women in the medical field and discovered that these women value quality in both their personal and their professional lives. These women strive to balance their careers with family, community, and extracurricular activities. The authors concluded that this finding is likely reflective of the more recent generations of physicians regardless of gender. However, such balance requires establishing an evolving set of priorities and, perhaps, patience in achieving career goals.

## Integrity

Personal integrity is essential for successful negotiations. A new faculty member's core values are regularly expressed in the daily tasks and interactions of academic life. The basic values of honesty, ethics, and professionalism are evidenced, as are other important variables such as the ability to collaborate with others, accept feedback and learn from mistakes, and positively relate to colleagues, students, and patients. Citizenship and collegiality are highly prized by senior faculty in leadership positions (see Chapter 26) (Boice 1992a; Raehl 2002).

Characteristics that earn junior faculty a negative appraisal from department chairs include negative attitude, lack of productivity, poor committee participation, social isolation, and lack of emotional regulation. Conversely, characteristics that engender trust and credibility include productivity, fulfilling commitments within the time expectation, participating in committees and task forces, attending department meetings, and maintaining a positive attitude regardless of the assignment. Individuals with exceptional careers meet all job expectations and find ways to make a positive impact beyond the job description (Citrin and Smith 2003). Essentially, the department chair appreciates faculty members who contribute to the department's mission and the school of medicine's success, even if it necessitates an ostensible pause in that faculty member's career goals.

## DEPARTMENTAL ATTRIBUTES

### Perspective

Each individual has a unique perspective through which he or she perceives and experiences the world. Likewise, institutions and their leaders have explicit and implicit assumptions that establish frames for expected behavior by the organization's members (see Chapter 10) (Cohen 2003; Russo and Schoemaker 2002; Seaman 1999). Understanding the department chair's beliefs, motives, and leadership style is imperative for successful negotiations. Mentors are valuable resources in this endeavor. An optimal mentor comprehends the department's politics and has a position of influence, respect from colleagues, and a commitment to advance the new faculty member's career (see Chapter 26).

Explicit or formal frames are found in the school of medicine's mission statement and promotion guidelines. Invariably, new faculty members are in concordance with these principles. Conflict may ensue if one's career trajectory changes without the support of leadership; for example, the faculty member's passion moves from research to clinical practice.

Implicit frames can be ascertained from observing and interacting with colleagues. A curious learner will acquire answers to important questions such as: Are junior faculty allowed to provide input into program and policy development? Does the department chair allow faculty to have autonomy in designated roles? From whom does the department chair accept meaningful feedback? Who among the faculty is respected? Who is involved in the decision-making processes for the department? What are the external forces that influence the department chair and the department?

Early career achievers actively engage senior and junior faculty to attain knowledge and guidance about the culture and values of the department (Boice 1992b; Raehl 2002). These early achievers also network with colleagues from outside their departments to better understand the context in which their departments function and to develop collaborative projects with other professionals.

### Finances

Negotiations cannot proceed until the financial terrain has been adequately mapped. Psychiatry departments receive funding from various sources, such as the parent university, endowments, state entities, research grants, partnerships with industry or hospitals, service contracts, and fees for service. Political or financial changes at any of the funding streams can radically affect a department's fiscal stability. The department chair's priorities and commitments are often contingent on the department's monetary resources. One of the chair's primary responsibilities is to maintain the department's operational status. Because schools of medicine and departments are increasingly required to operate within a balanced budget, requests for new funding demand additional justification. Certain obligations, such as base salaries, cannot be compromised; however, new projects or nonessential projects can be placed on hold or discontinued. Knowing how to secure or access funding for a new proposal is mandatory.

## NEGOTIATIONS

Now that the culture of the department is appreciated and faculty credibility has been established, direct negotiations and self-advocacy can begin. Though the term may be an overused one, a "win-win" situation is the objective of successful negotiation. Cohen (2003) notes that "negotiation in the final analysis requires two parties to say yes" (p. 11). Both the junior faculty and the department chair say yes because each benefits from the negotiated agreement. Arriving at an agreement demands thorough preparation, awareness of the power differential, access to funding, alignment with the department's goals, and a steady focus.

### Power Differential

Recognition of the power differential between the department chair and the faculty member is an absolute prerequisite to the negotiation process. Not only does the department chair have assigned authority but also, by virtue of this appointment, a record of successful negotiations. Attempts to establish a sense of power by controlling the discussion, minimizing the department chair's input, or challenging his or her authority and expertise in any way will likely lead to a premature cessation of the negotiating process. Qualities such as respect, active listening, and modesty will maintain the process.

Acceptance of the power differential does not imply a position of passivity. Instead, it encourages courteous assertiveness. Respectful engagement allows for active dialogue and flexible problem solving. The department chair will present vital perspectives that the faculty member may not have considered. Of course, the dialogue is more constructive if an interpersonal relationship has already been established. Though a positive relationship advances the negotiation process, it is still important to maintain emotional distance during the actual negotiations. Too much emotionality can impair the ability to incorporate information and maintain focus.

Power also resides in the capacity to take risks, adhere to values, and maintain a vision—but only if the faculty member has credibility. There is also power in the ability to be patient and persistent. At the University of New Mexico, an associate who is credited as an effective negotiator is described as "a steady stream of water that erodes the rocks."

## Finances

One must be equipped with the information and financial data to support a proposal. Data that are presented in a manner that is congruent with the department chair's preferences is more likely to be assimilated. Does the chair want graphs and spread sheets, a detailed written report on all the possible outcomes, or a brief summary with bullet points?

Presentation of the finances encompasses a delineation of the project's cost in terms of materials and human resources, the source of funding, and the effect on the department's budget. Also included is the breakdown of the indirect and overhead costs. For example, a service contract with a local school system must cover the faculty member's salary and the costs of benefits (e.g., health insurance), administrative support, supplies, and travel time. Another component is calculating the availability of other faculty to perform the work that is left unattended while the school contract is being executed.

## Congruency

Proposals that are aligned with the department and school of medicine's purpose and mission have a higher probability of being approved. Moreover, proposals that are congruent with external stakeholders' expectations and demands will be viewed more favorably. These stakeholders include university administrators, accreditation and regulatory agencies, consumer and advocacy groups, funding sources, research partners from other universities and government offices, and clinical community partners. For instance, a state agency prioritizes treatment for substance abuse and attaches funding for the university for the delivery of these services. An observant faculty member with a commitment to this clinical work will be ready with a plan that allows for protected time to develop and implement a substance abuse program.

Ideally, the faculty member has consulted with mentors and senior colleagues to determine the viability of the proposition. Senior associates can assess the value of an idea in both monetary and nonmonetary ways. An initiative's value may reside in the new opportunities or innovations it creates, the status it brings, or the problems it solves for the department. The willingness to accept critical feedback from esteemed colleagues helps strengthen the proposal and one's ability to negotiate with the department chair. If the initial negotiation does not yield the desired results, rethink the process. Integrate the feedback into the formulation, consult with senior colleagues, realign the proposal to the department's mission, know how to access the funding, renew the vision and passion, and be prepared to be a steady stream.

# CASE SCENARIOS

## Scenario 1

A junior faculty member wants to develop an evidence-based, community-based treatment program for children who are at risk for out-of-home placement. This program will positively position the department for future negotiations with a state managed care system.

**Option A:** Faculty member talks to department chair and explains the benefits of the program; requests protected time to develop it. Department chair's response: due to financial pressures, the faculty member needs to remain with the current assignment and reach productivity expectations.

**Option B:** Faculty member, on his or her own time and with leadership's knowledge, discusses project with interested stakeholders to determine if there is genuine interest in the program. Consumer groups and managed care system provide positive response. Faculty member works with administrators to do cost analysis and financial impact on department, develops proposal that shows a profit, and presents to department chair. Department chair's response: assigns division director to project to work with faculty member to initiate its development.

## Scenario 2

An early career psychiatrist wants to change focus from treatment to research. Specifically, she wants to develop a research site for posttraumatic stress disorder.

**Option A:** Faculty member asks to be transferred to outpatient clinic to provide outpatient services and develop a research protocol. Department chair's response: offers faculty member the opportunity to change positions with a hospital-based psychiatrist who also wants a change; also offers faculty member a 10% incentive to do inpatient work. Chair needs for both psychiatrists to deliver patient care due to contract obligations.

**Option B:** Faculty member collaborates, on his or her own time, with internal and external colleagues to submit a research grant to federal funding source. Asks department chair for protected time if grant is funded for at least 3 years. Department chair's response: will grant protected time if grant is funded.

## SMART STRATEGIES

- Establish a personal purpose and mission that is based on passion and that is larger than the individual.
- Maintain personal integrity.
- Contribute to the department's mission and success.
- Understand the department's finances and know how to access funding for the new proposal; understand the financial impact of the proposal.
- Recognize the power that the department chair possesses.
- Communicate the value of the proposal.
- Create a win-win transaction through creative problem solving.

## QUESTIONS TO DISCUSS WITH A MENTOR OR COLLEAGUE

1. How have you achieved career satisfaction?
2. How does an early career faculty member demonstrate competence and credibility in the department?
3. What are the implicit faculty qualities that are valued by the department?
4. How is the early career faculty member's purpose aligned with the department's?
5. What are the internal forces (e.g., school of medicine) and the external forces (e.g., state agencies) that affect the department?

## REFERENCES

Boice R: Chair-faculty relations. Academic Leader 7:1–2, 1992a
Boice R: The New Faculty Member. San Francisco, CA, Jossey-Bass, 1992b

Brown AJ, Swinyard W, Ogle J: Women in academic medicine: a report of focus groups and questionnaires, with conjoint analysis. J Womens Health 12:999–1008, 2003

Citrin JS, Smith RA: The 5 Patterns of Extraordinary Careers. New York, Crown Business, 2003

Cohen H: Negotiate This. New York, Warner Books, 2003

Raehl CL: Changes in pharmacy practice faculty 1995–2001: implications for junior faculty development. Pharmacotherapy 22:445–462, 2002

Russo JE, Schoemaker PJH: Winning Decisions: Getting It Right the First Time. New York, Doubleday, 2002

Seaman R: The Path. Palo Alto, CA, Guidance Press, 1999

## ADDITIONAL RESOURCES

Fisher R, Ury W: Getting to Yes: Negotiating Agreement Without Giving In, 2nd Edition. New York, Penguin Books, 1981

# CHAPTER 13

# Developing Your Ethics Skills

Ryan Spellecy, Ph.D.

Laura Weiss Roberts, M.D., M.A.

Psychiatrists are often called on to help resolve knotty problems. These problems may arise in clinical, educational, research, or administrative activities, and they may be ethical in nature. Psychiatrists may also serve as members of ethics committees, institutional review boards, academic progress committees, peer review groups, and policy-making bodies that carry the responsibility for ethical decision making within academic settings. Psychiatrists may be particularly well suited to this work because of the focused attention the profession gives to communication, clarity, and contextual issues. Nevertheless, it is valuable to have specific knowledge and a suite of skills for ethical problem solving in these diverse potential roles of the academic psychiatrist.

The aim of this chapter is to outline key ethics skills as well as to characterize ethical and legal standards in psychiatric practice with regard to informed consent, advance directives and alternative decision-makers, and confidentiality.

## ETHICS SKILLS

### Skill 1: Identification

The ability to arrive at and enact ethically sound decisions involves a specific set of skills (Roberts 2003; Roberts and Dyer 2004; Jonsen et al.

1986). The first and often most important of these skills is the ability to identify ethically important and values-laden aspects of a professional situation. Recognizing ethical issues in the care of a person whose decisional capacity is compromised and who refuses life-saving treatment is not difficult. However, it is much harder to see the full set of ethical issues that may accompany the care of a medical student who seeks treatment at his or her training institution or the care of a person with schizophrenia who prefers oral medication to depot administration but has been unable to remain adherent to his or her treatment plan. Even more challenging are the ethical issues associated with a faculty member evaluating protocols of an investigator in an adjacent laboratory for the institutional review board (IRB): the reviewer possesses the expertise needed but may compete with the colleague for resources or institutional status. This first skill involves being sensitive to situations and noting when something may not be quite right as a marker of a possible ethical problem.

## Skill 2: Information Gathering

The second skill is the ability to gather information that may help to shed light on the ethical features of the professional situation. Important resources related to this skill include scholarly literature, institutional policies, experts in the given field, and stakeholders in the situation. Literature resources can vary from conceptual or theoretical ethics to empirical studies concerning specific ethical issues or topics, their scope, incidence, and more. Purely theoretical literature may be of little use or may be difficult to apply to clinical practice, and empirical literature concerning ethics make unjustified theoretical assumptions, which raises questions concerning its validity. The most useful literature has a strong conceptual background but is informed by clinical observation and empirical research.

Persons with expertise in ethics, law, and cultural and religious issues represent other potential resources. Many institutions have at least one person serving on their ethics committee with expertise in ethics. An ethics committee can also refer you to any policies that have ethical relevance, and an IRB will have experts familiar with ethical issues in research. Of course, lawyers are excellent resources for specific legal issues in your jurisdiction, such as advance directives, surrogate decision making, or civil commitment. Finally, stakeholders (consumer advocacy groups, family members, etc.) and social workers are often quite savvy concerning legal and ethical issues in psychiatry.

## Skill 3: Application of Principles

A third ethics skill is the ability to clarify and apply relevant principles of the profession to the situation. Principlism is one widely accepted approach in clinical ethics that provides guidance through identifying and considering four ethical principles in particular: autonomy, beneficence, nonmaleficence, and justice (Beauchamp and Childress 2001).

The application of these concepts is not especially straightforward, however. For instance, autonomy is the most familiar principle, yet is often misunderstood. Autonomy is a rich, nuanced ideal pertaining to liberty, the capacity for deliberation, and information. It does not mean, as some assume, that caregivers are required to accede to patient wishes. If a patient states a wish that stems from false information, his or her decisional abilities may be impaired, or if coercive pressures are perceived in the environment, honoring the wish would *not* technically respect that patient's autonomy (Roberts 2002). Beneficence, or "doing good," exhorts us to maximize the benefits for our patients. It is important to temper beneficence with other principles to avoid paternalism, which is defined as interfering with someone's liberty for his or her own perceived good, regardless of the individual's preferences. Nonmaleficence is captured by the maxim "do no harm." This is sometimes confused with beneficence, but it differs in that it requires us to avoid unnecessary harm to patients. What constitutes unnecessary harm? Autonomy or beneficence, when balanced against nonmaleficence, could surely render harm necessary to achieve an important goal. For example, the side effects of a medication, though considered a harm, might be outweighed by a patient's desire to manage his or her symptoms. Justice (distributive or social justice) is the final and least discussed principle. Used in the context of bioethics, justice refers to the distribution of goods and burdens in society. Questions of justice are central to issues such as treatment of the uninsured and underinsured, managed care, and mental health parity for insurance coverage.

Other bioethics concepts such as veracity, integrity, compassion, and respect for the law are also of vital importance in clarifying ethical considerations. In the practice of psychiatry, key ethics issues commonly arise in relation to the principles of privacy (the right to control one's personal information), confidentiality (refraining from sharing knowledge of another's personal information), and veracity (truth telling), which can be traced to concerns for autonomy, beneficence, nonmaleficence, and perhaps even justice, depending on the clinical circumstances. The importance of principlism for psychiatrists lies in its ability to classify ethical issues in clinical practice and its dependence upon balancing these principles when they conflict.

## Skill 4: Decision Making

Being able to recognize, seek a greater understanding of, and clarify ethical aspects of a professional situation are followed by the fourth skill of exploring and weighing the choices at hand through a systematic decision-making model. There are several meritorious approaches to decision making. One common model for clinical ethics decision making is illustrated in Figure 13–1. The various decision-making models all focus on the importance of having a clear rationale for a course of action and being explicit about decisions that are governed by certain principles above others (e.g., a decision to place compassion, beneficence, nonmaleficence, and adherence with the law above autonomy when placing a seriously ill and dangerous patient on an involuntary hold) when a dilemma or conflict exists.

## Skill 5: Taking Action and Remaining Vigilant

The fifth skill involves taking deliberate action in a manner that involves multiple safeguards to help you remain vigilant to unintended consequences and to minimize harms that may be associated with a particular decision. Safeguards include 1) collaboration with colleagues in enacting the decision; 2) engaging in vigorous self-observation; 3) inviting in "critical friends" to help with subsequent decision making; 4) creating checkpoints to evaluate the positive and negative aspects of a decision; 5) finding ways to undertake midcourse corrections in light of worsening outcomes, new information, unexpected challenges, or problems; and 6) debriefing after a decision has played out. This series of steps allows for 1) action, 2) control and correction of consequences, 3) collaboration and "buy in" from individuals who otherwise may not understand and possibly may undermine your decisions in a hard situation, 4) and learning so that the next situation might not be so hard.

## INFORMED CONSENT

Informed consent has emerged as a clinical, ethical, and legal standard important to the practice of every physician. For every treatment decision or research enrollment decision, the physician and patient should engage in a careful informed consent process. The primary ethical prin-

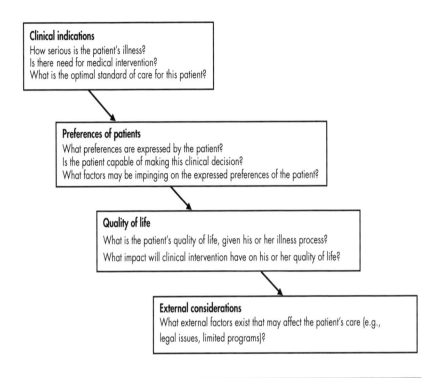

**FIGURE 13–1.** Clinical ethics decision-making model.

*Source.* From Roberts LW, Dunn LB: "Ethical Considerations in Caring for Women With Substance Use Disorders." *Obstetrics and Gynecology Clinics of North America* 30:559–582, 2003. Reprinted with permission from Elsevier.

ciple involved is respect for autonomy. Because the individual giving his or her consent must ultimately live with the consequences of that decision, he or she must truly understand the decision and make it freely. Additionally, since issues of risk and benefit have subjective elements that vary in degree from person to person, a competent individual is best able to consider risks and benefits against his or her own values, desires, goals, and beliefs.

The three elements that comprise informed consent, as illustrated in Figure 13–2, are 1) the sharing of information; 2) the decisional capacity of the patient, study participant, or his or her representative; and 3) the capacity for voluntarism (Appelbaum and Grisso 1988). In Figure 13–2, "information" involves the sharing of information in a manner that fosters an autonomous decision on the part of the patient. The concept of fostering an autonomous decision is important, because either too little *or* too much information might detract from one's capacity to decide and act autonomously. Although it is not possible to list the information required for informed consent in all situations, general information regarding the illness, likely risks and benefits, procedures involved in the proposed treatment, alternatives to the recommended treatment (including no treatment), and expected outcomes are all good places to start. Additionally, the "reasonable patient standard," which states that informed consent requires that you share the information that a reasonable patient who is similarly situated would want to know, is a good guideline to consider.

Another useful tool for thinking about the informative aspects of informed consent is the transparency model (Brody 1989). This model states that an individual has sufficient information when the physician has made a recommendation and has rendered transparent to the patient the reasoning behind the physician's choice of that recommendation. This may require explaining why one intervention was recommended as opposed to others, what risks and benefits were relevant to the decision, the suspected outcomes of various interventions, and so on. By explaining his or her thought process associated with the recommended treatment in accessible terms to the individual, the physician has executed the "informed" element of informed consent.

The second element of informed consent, decisional capacity, is the ability to evaluate and appreciate the information as it relates to the individual. There are four constituent components to decisional capacity. The first component is the individual's ability to express a preference. This is relatively straightforward, but bear in mind that individuals may express preferences through different mediums (consider patients with dysphasia), and it is your responsibility to find a medium that enables your patients to do so. The second component is the ability to understand relevant information, such as the nature of the illness, prognosis, risks, benefits, and alternatives to the proposed intervention. The third component is the ability to reason. This requires that the patient be able to make logical connections, such as understanding causes and effects of treatments and decisions. Additionally, if two treatments promise the same benefits, although one has greater risks and side effects, a rational person will choose the less risky treatment. The fourth component of informed consent, and often most difficult to evaluate because it involves subjective elements, is the individual's ability to appreciate the information and its relevance to his or her own goals, desires, life plans, experiences, and other issues.

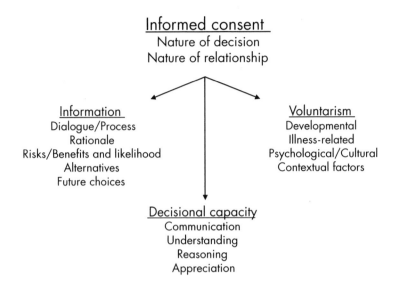

Informed consent
Nature of decision
Nature of relationship

Information
Dialogue/Process
Rationale
Risks/Benefits and likelihood
Alternatives
Future choices

Voluntarism
Developmental
Illness-related
Psychological/Cultural
Contextual factors

Decisional capacity
Communication
Understanding
Reasoning
Appreciation

**FIGURE 13–2.** Key elements of informed consent.

*Source.* Adapted from Roberts LW, Dyer AR: "Informed Consent and Decisional Capacity" in *Concise Guide to Ethics in Mental Health Care*. Washington, DC, American Psychiatric Publishing, 2004, p. 52. Used with permission.

It is widely accepted that decisional capacity requirements should be seen as a risk-relative sliding scale. This means that as the risk associated with accepting or refusing a course of treatment increases, so too does the stringency of the standard for competency (Drane 1985). For example, in a scenario involving a potentially dangerous treatment, or if there is a range of alternative treatments, an individual must demonstrate the ability to understand the outcomes of the various treatments, balance risks and benefits, and make a decision on this basis. If the risk increases, such as in a life-threatening decision, an individual must not only understand the medical information but also how it applies to his or her life, values, and goals. As Drane (1985) explains, "The competent patient must be able to give reasons for the decision, which show that he has thought through the medical issues and related this information to his personal values" (p. 20). A simple example might be that the evaluation of decision-making capacity to consent for a routine blood test would be less stringent than it would for a decision to refuse life-sustaining medical treatment. It is worth noting that this model can yield the conclusion that decisional capacity should be more stringently evaluated for the refusal of some treatments than for the acceptance of those same treatments, if refusal carries significantly greater risk.

The final element of informed consent is the capacity for voluntarism. Voluntarism refers to the individual's ability to act in accord with his or her authentic sense of what is good, right, and best in light of his or her situation, values, and history (Roberts 2002). Voluntarism further entails the capacity to make a choice freely and in the absence of coercion. Deliberateness, purposefulness of intent, clarity, genuineness, and coherence with prior life decisions are implicitly emphasized. Coherence with prior life decisions is particularly interesting, as it enables one to consider the values of a person over time, giving a richer understanding of autonomy.

The capacity for voluntariness should be systematically assessed along four dimensions: 1) developmental factors, 2) illness-related considerations, 3) psychological issues and cultural and religious values, and 4) external pressures. Developmental factors include youth or developmental disabilities that interfere with the generation of personal values and the capacity for autonomous choice. Illness-related considerations include symptoms such as the negative cognitive distortions and hopelessness associated with depression or the amotivation associated with addiction or psychotic disorders. Psychological issues include the expectations and perceptions of the individual. Cultural and religious values may affect an individual's sense of personal agency in relation to the greater authority that may exist within his or her family or spiritual community. External pressures, such as institutionalization or poverty, may diminish the individual's sense of power and voluntarism. Finally, it is important to note that the presence of any or all of these dimensions would not necessarily eliminate or even severely impair the capacity for voluntarism.

Before we leave informed consent, there are two final important remarks to consider. Informed consent is *not* the document that the patient signs. Obviously, a patient can sign that document without meeting any of the above elements. Additionally, informed consent is not a one-time event, but rather is an ongoing process. Each time you see a patient or research participant, the informed consent dialogue should continue. Are there newly identified risks or benefits for the intervention? Perhaps your patient is experiencing side effects that give him or her a new perspective on the treatments that needs to be weighed in terms of his or her values. Any number of issues can arise over the course of treatment (or a study) that necessitate an ongoing dialogue of informed consent.

## ADVANCE DIRECTIVES AND ALTERNATIVE DECISION-MAKERS

When a person is not capable of making a health-related decision in our society, other means may be employed that seek to uphold the prior autonomous choices of the patient. These means include advance directives (both living wills and power of attorney for health care documents) and surrogate decision-makers. We will discuss the various mechanisms in descending order, or beginning with the mechanisms that are closest to informed consent.

Advance directives are legal documents that seek to enable us to make decisions as the patient would have wanted. A living will is a written statement of treatment preferences, whereas a power of attorney for health care allows the patient to appoint someone to make decisions on his or her behalf during periods of decisional incapacity (sometimes with written directions from the patient to guide the power of attorney). The benefit of a living will is that when thoroughly written, it provides explicit instructions from the patient. However, no one can envision all circumstances in which one might find oneself, thereby limiting the usefulness of the guidance contained in the document. The benefit of a power of attorney for health care is that the person appointed by the document can make decisions based on the values of the patient; it thereby offers more flexibility than a living will, although making a decision based on someone else's complex value system is a difficult task.

If a nondecisional patient does not have an advance directive, the next best choice is a surrogate decision-maker who is familiar with the patient's values, wishes, and goals. Ethically, there may be little difference between a surrogate who knows the patient and a person granted power of attorney by the patient, but legally they are distinct. Finally, if there is no advance directive and no one willing or able to serve as a surrogate, the courts may appoint a guardian. Although a court-appointed guardian can and should still attempt to make decisions in accord with the wishes of the patient, or using "substituted judgment," sometimes a "best interests" standard must be used, in which the guardian endeavors to make decisions that an informed, reasonable person would make.

All of these approaches are ethical as well as legal mechanisms, so their implementation will vary from state to state. In some states, there is a statutorily defined order of preference for surrogates (spouse, then adult children, then parents, etc.); other states have no such statutes. A mentor will be able not only to clarify such legal issues but also to aid you in using these mechanisms to best honor patient autonomy without sacrificing beneficence and nonmaleficence.

## CONFIDENTIALITY

Confidentiality is an implicit promise that is "present when one person discloses information to another, whether through words or an examination, and the person to whom the information is disclosed pledges not to divulge that information to a third party without the confider's permission" (Beauchamp 2001, p. 305). Ethically, it is a duty of nondisclosure that "necessarily involves another party with whom private information is shared on the basis of trust" (Wettstein 1994, p. 344). The aspect of trust is important to consider in psychiatry because breaking confidentiality can harm the therapeutic relationship.

Although autonomy is the dominant principle here, nonmaleficence is also at stake because divulging personal information can harm a patient's personal and professional relationships. While confidentiality is as old as medical ethics itself, having found its way into the Hippocratic oath (Miles 2004), it is not inviolable. Legal requirements that allow or even require (duty to warn) the violation of confidentiality vary from state to state (Jones 2003). Some examples that would justify breaking confidentiality are danger to self or others; abuse of children, elders, or others with compromised decisional capacity; and, in some jurisdictions, informing partners or a government entity such as the health department of a person's HIV status (Herbert and Young 2002; Huprich et al. 2003). When appropriate, informing patients at the beginning of treatment of the conditions that might require violating confidentiality can mitigate future problems.

Regardless of the situations in which the law might permit or require the violation of confidentiality, the ethical considerations behind these statutes involve a weighing of the autonomy and welfare (beneficence) of the patient versus potential harm (nonmaleficence). Even though the severity and probability of harm might justify violating confidentiality, one should still seek any avenues short of violating confidentiality whenever possible. However, if breaking confidentiality becomes necessary, actions should be chosen that preserve it as much as possible. Balancing the autonomy and welfare of your patient against potential harm to self or others is difficult. Asking a mentor for advice and suggestions in this area is certainly prudent.

## SMART STRATEGIES

- Make a concerted effort to develop your ethics skill set.
  - Sharpen sensitivity to ethically important and values-laden aspects of a professional situation.

- Gather information through a literature search, identification of stakeholders, and a thorough review of institutional policies when confronted with an ethical question.
- Clarify and apply relevant principles of the profession to the ethics situation.
- Explore and weigh the choices at hand through a systematic decision-making model.
- Take deliberate action in a manner that involves multiple safeguards to minimize harm.

- Seek out the expertise and guidance of colleagues and consultants to help with ethics issues as they arise.
- Learn more about the interdependence of clinical, legal, and ethical aspects of your professional work.

## QUESTIONS TO DISCUSS WITH A MENTOR OR COLLEAGUE

1. What ethics resources are available at my institution? Is there an ethics center?
2. Whom can I contact from the IRB for questions regarding the ethical conduct of research?
3. Whom can I contact from the hospital ethics committee if I have questions concerning clinical ethics? Is there an ethics consulting service for the hospital, and if so, how do I request a consultation?
4. Who are some of the stakeholders in the community, such as advocacy groups?
5. What are the regulatory issues that are relevant to my locality concerning advance directives, determining a surrogate decision-maker, the duty to warn, and the like?

## REFERENCES

Appelbaum PS, Grisso T: Assessing patients' capacities to consent to treatment. N Engl J Med 319:1635–1638, 1988

Beauchamp TL, Childress JF: Principles of Biomedical Ethics, 5th Edition. New York, Oxford University Press, 2001

Brody H: Transparency: informed consent in primary care. Hastings Cent Rep 19:5–9, 1989

Drane JF: The many faces of competency. Hastings Cent Rep 15:17–21, 1985

Herbert PB, Young KA: *Tarasoff* at twenty-five. J Am Acad Psychiatry Law 30:275–281, 2002

Huprich SK, Fuller KM, Schneider RB: Divergent ethical perspectives on the duty-to-warn principle with HIV patients. Ethics Behav 13:263–278, 2003

Jones C: Tightropes and tragedies: 25 years of Tarasoff. Med Sci Law 43:13–22, 2003

Jonsen AR, Siegler M, Winslade WJ: Clinical Ethics: A Practical Approach to Ethical Decisions in Clinical Medicine, 2nd Edition. New York, Macmillan, 1986

Miles S: The Hippocratic Oath and the Ethics of Medicine. Oxford, Oxford University Press, 2004

Roberts LW: Informed consent and the capacity for voluntarism. Am J Psychiatry 159:705–712, 2002

Roberts LW: Ethical principles and skills in the care of mental illness. Focus 1:339–344, 2003

Roberts LW, Dyer AR: Concise Guide to Ethics in Mental Health Care. Washington, DC, American Psychiatric Publishing, 2004

Wettstein R: Confidentiality. Review of Psychiatry 13:343–364, 1994

## ADDITIONAL RESOURCES

Edwards RB: Ethics of Psychiatry: Insanity, Rational Autonomy and Mental Health Care. Amherst, NY, Prometheus Books, 1997

Hundert EM: A model for ethical problem solving in medicine, with practical applications. Am J Psychiatry 144:839–846, 1987

# PART IV

# Becoming an Educator...

# CHAPTER 14

# Giving Feedback

### Jon Lehrmann, M.D.

> [Feedback is] information that a system uses to
> make adjustments in reaching a goal.
>
> *Jack Ende*

Feedback is essential to learning. It is one element of an iterative, interactive process that allows for the growth, strengthening, and enhancement of valuable traits and knowledge. It is a concept that is, at its core, rather mechanical and nonjudgmental; feedback is the way in which a system changes its "general methods and pattern of performance" by "reinserting into the system the results of its performance" (Ende 1983, p. 177). Positive feedback exerts a stimulatory, amplifying effect on a key step of a system, whereas negative feedback exerts an inhibitory, diminishing effect on a key step of a system. Feedback often has an observational, here-and-now focus, and it may not carry as much of a value judgment as other forms of performance evaluation.

Accurate, constructive, and compassionately delivered feedback to a learner is a gift (see Chapter 26). We learn more effectively if we can change and try alternative methods immediately upon receiving information—when we can directly tie together the cause and effect. Knowing how to give feedback and how to help learners find ways to improve their performance is a sophisticated skill, one that is seldom taught. It may come more naturally for some faculty members than others, but it is one that should be both rehearsed and practiced. In this chapter, we outline forms of feedback, give examples of common missteps related to giving feedback, and provide tips for giving feedback.

## FORMS OF FEEDBACK

Feedback can be nonverbal or verbal. It can be positive or negative, but it shouldn't be equated with compliments or criticisms. Every expression and body posture we make, even the timing of our actions, may be observed, interpreted, and experienced by those around us. This nonverbal communication is a form of feedback, and it can have a great impact. Being self-observing of one's posture and nonverbal cues is extremely valuable. Sometimes psychiatrists struggle with assessing their countertransferential feelings. Paying attention to your muscle tension, posture, and nonverbal behavior can help you better know your inner feelings. Some of the most important learning experiences in becoming a psychiatrist include doing mock board examination exercises and being videotaped to see one's physical style in interacting with others.

Positive verbal feedback can be especially powerful. For instance, the clinical supervisor who comments, "Paying attention to the patient's affect as you did is very important in developing rapport" during bedside teaching rounds can have a very encouraging effect on a student. Positive verbal feedback is naturally supportive of the positive motivations of individuals who want to do things well and correctly and who wish to develop and grow. To illustrate this point, a presenter at a business leadership seminar asked for feedback and then stood at a whiteboard and began to do some basic math problems. She added 7 plus 7 and wrote down the sum of 14. She wrote 9 plus 8 and wrote the sum of 17. The room was quiet. She wrote 9 plus 3 equals 12 and then 7 plus 5 equals 11. Eight people raised their hands and several spoke out, "That should be 12." She turned around and smiled. She asked the group to notice that she had asked for feedback, but that only when she made a mistake did she get a response. Most of us grow up and develop in a system where negative feedback or criticism is the norm and positive feedback is rarely given. For these reasons, it is especially important to be attentive and proactive in looking for opportunities to give positive feedback as well as negative feedback. When feedback is commonplace and is offered in the right spirit, this effort will be seen as a gift and will improve morale.

A compliment is not the same as positive feedback. A compliment is an interpersonal exchange that seeks to make someone feel better. "You are great" is an example of a compliment. A compliment may provide information, but positive feedback will be more specific and aims to improve performance.

Negative feedback is specific information given in a neutral, supportive manner with the intent to help someone improve performance. Negative feedback is not intended to influence or directly affect the feelings of the learner. For example, a common mistake in the Mini-Mental State Examination is when a student has a patient do serial sevens to test concentration and recurrently reminds the patient of the task before every subtraction. When this is witnessed, negative feedback, such as "Reminding the patient of the task recurrently is really only testing the patient's ability to subtract and does not measure her ability to attend to and concentrate on the task," is appropriate and should help the student learn how to correctly assess concentration.

Criticism is not the same as negative feedback. Criticism tends to be more general, and it may have the primary objective of making the person giving the criticism feel better and the recipient of the criticism feel worse. Criticism in the above example might be something like, "You don't even know how to do the simple task of testing concentration."

## COMMON MISSTEPS RELATED TO FEEDBACK

There are several potential "missteps" related to giving feedback (Table 14–1). A common mistake is to withhold feedback because there is concern that feelings will be hurt. When negative feedback is not given, a pattern of errors or problems may emerge, and this does not serve the interests or needs of the student. Moreover, most students would rather get the negative feedback (in a nonshaming, nonthreatening way) than receive none at all and continue to make the same mistakes. Those who deliver negative feedback, despite the anxiety about doing so that they may experience, are usually relieved on finding that it was not nearly as bad as was feared. Negative feedback does not usually lead to conflict—especially if the feedback is given in a caring and supportive way. Even giving positive feedback can feel awkward. Worrying about how the feedback is interpreted is a common concern.

Interjecting demeaning comments while working with students can hurt feelings and make a supervision traumatic experience for them. There is never a situation when this should be done. Supervisors and teachers need to be aware of their own feelings (especially anger) and do whatever is necessary to prevent the anger from coming out in a demeaning way. However, this does not mean that supervisors cannot communicate their frustration.

**TABLE 14–1.**    Feedback missteps

| Common misstep | Correction | Example |
|---|---|---|
| Avoiding giving feedback because it is too time-intensive or awkward. | Taking time now saves time later, and if done in a diplomatic and caring way, it will not be awkward. | "Let's be sure to set some time aside later this week to talk through your write-ups." |
| Interjecting demeaning or personal comments. ("You are the slowest resident I have ever worked with.") | Keep your personal feelings about the student out of the feedback. | "Your pace during the interview and presentation was slow. I'd like to see you pick up the pace a bit next time." |
| Confusing praise with positive feedback. ("Your write-up was awesome—you really are great.") | Be objective with positive feedback, and leave personal comments out. | "I felt the MSE in your write-up was nicely organized and complete." |
| Confusing criticism with negative feedback. ("Only a stupid resident would release him.") | Be objective with negative feedback. | "Were you aware that we keep the old records over here? It is essential that we take the time to review the old records prior to deciding the disposition." |
| Not being objective enough. ("You did a great job.") | Have objective methods to measure and evaluate prior to the occurrence of teaching interactions and apply them. | "Your biopsychosocial formulation was very complete, but ECT would have been another biological treatment option to have included." |
| Giving feedback in front of peers. | Especially when giving negative feedback, take the student aside away from peers or patients. | A daily time set at the end of rounds to meet with each student for 5–10 minutes to give feedback would help eliminate this problem. |
| Only giving negative feedback. | Look for opportunities to give positive feedback. It takes extra effort, but is worth it. | "I like the way you introduced yourself to the patient." |

It is a common misstep to give praise instead of or as part of feedback. Most educators want to be liked by their students and want their students to feel good about themselves. Giving praise often makes a student feel good and the supervisor feel benevolent, but it may distort the goal of the situation: the student is there to learn! Positive performance by the student should naturally be viewed positively by the supervisor, but the primary goal of the interaction is not pleasing the teacher but professional growth and development of the learner.

Using criticism instead of negative feedback is another misstep, and it can be personally devastating to the learner. An example of some particularly painful criticism was a comment made by an attending physician to a first-year resident on rotation to the psychiatric emergency room. The resident had evaluated a suicidal patient and was presenting the case to the supervising attending physician. The resident was leaning toward releasing the patient from the clinical setting back to his home. The attending had reviewed records that the resident did not know existed that indicated a significantly increased risk for suicide. The attending stated in front of all the other residents there, "Only a stupid doctor would let the patient go without reviewing all the records." The resident was hurt and embarrassed. Negative feedback was definitely required, but a much better way to address this serious situation with the resident would have been to ask the resident if all the records had been thoroughly reviewed. (In this case, the new resident had not known where old records were kept and had not seen them.) If the resident had not seen all of the records, the proper guidance would have been to have the resident review them and only then recommend a disposition. If the resident still was not considering suicide risk appropriately, negative feedback would be further indicated.

One of the most common missteps in feedback is lack of objectivity. Usually, this is because time is not taken in advance to review objective measures. Supervisors often learn what will be evaluated ahead of time, and it is to their benefit to have set, objective measures and goals by which to evaluate. If there are not preexisting standards to guide measurement, then creating some usually can be done fairly easily; for example, create a checklist to assess an interview's completeness. Taking this approach requires more work up front, but the value of the feedback is increased tenfold.

Sometimes, although not always, giving feedback in front of a group can be a misstep. Feedback is best given individually when possible. Even positive feedback in front of peers can be embarrassing—students still call each other "gunners" (a term used to describe competitive students who try to impress their supervisors, often with the intention of making their colleagues look worse by comparison). Still, some business leaders feel giving positive feedback in front of peers is a powerful way to encourage a positive atmosphere. More effort should be given to providing negative feedback in a one-on-one format.

A final common misstep is not giving enough positive feedback and giving negative feedback more often. People tend not to notice as much and not to give feedback when things are done right. When things go wrong, it is common to scrutinize and to try to get things on track. It is natural to give negative feedback, but doing so exclusively is insufficient in supporting the learning process.

## GIVING FEEDBACK

Are you giving feedback with the content and style you want? Many of us actively avoid giving feedback because it takes too much time and makes us uncomfortable, or because we feel the recipient will not take it well or read it correctly. Psychiatrists need to develop expertise in giving feedback. An important part of choosing what feedback to give is knowing and understanding who you are giving feedback to. Learning psychodynamic psychotherapy helps us better predict how feedback might be received and therefore can help us know and plan how best to give feedback without too much defensiveness developing on the part of the patient. Below are some helpful tips on how best to give feedback.

1. *Set up expectations and objectives for the learner* and determine your evaluation criteria in advance. This could be called "feedforward" (Whitman et al. 1993). This helps the learner and the teacher better define what is to be learned, how it will be assessed, and how feedback will be given.
2. *Encourage self-assessment.* Having the learner do a self-evaluation prior to your giving feedback can be extremely helpful. It will give you essential information about the learner's insight and risk of becoming defensive. If there is a significant gap between the learner's self-evaluation and your evaluation, it will be important to understand why.
3. *Foster a two-way feedback system.* Let the learner know that you will be giving feedback and the intervals in which it will be given. Ask to receive feedback from the learner as well. We can only improve ourselves with feedback. This can also help make the learner get better at giving feedback.

4. *Take the time to assess objectively;* create an objective system from which to measure. Know what your "ruler" is. What exactly are you measuring? To avoid subjective feedback such as "You did a great interview," you need to know what you are measuring ahead of time. What does that feedback really mean? How did the interviewer introduce herself? Did she establish rapport? How can you measure this? Did she deal with the patient's emotions effectively? Did she gather the information that was necessary in an efficient way? How was it rated? What exactly is a great interview? It would be much more valuable for the resident to be given specific examples objectively measured with regard to what was done right and what could be improved. There really is no such thing as a perfect interview.

5. *Minimize defensiveness:* don't point. In couples therapy we are taught to use "I" statements—not "you" statements. Present yourself as "happy, and with humility." Happy in that you are not angry with the person you are reviewing, humble in that you are not better or smarter than that person. A former colleague refers to this as the "Columbo approach," referring to Peter Falk's television character, a detective who confronted his suspects in a very nonthreatening way that did not elicit defensiveness. (For instance, he would scratch his forehead, looking confused, and ask the suspect how he could have been home at the time of the crime when a video shows him being at the bank.) In this approach, feedback—even negative feedback—can be given while minimizing the recipient's defensiveness to improve the chances that he or she will be able to actually listen and contemplate the feedback offered.

6. *Pay attention to your nonverbal communication.* Sit down if possible, especially if negative feedback is to be given. Use an open position (do not cross your arms). Provide good eye contact.

7. *Make sure you are giving sufficient positive feedback.* When it becomes necessary to give negative feedback, try to give some positive feedback first. This can also minimize defensiveness and allow the receiver to hear the feedback, especially if it is negative.

8. *Do not delay.* Timing is critical; the closer the feedback is chronologically to the behavior, the better. However, it is not possible to give immediate feedback in some settings, such as in a review of process notes or in the middle of a mock boards interview.

9. *Give the feedback face to face if possible.* Schum et al. (2003) found that learners preferred to receive feedback face to face or in written form rather than by e-mail.

10. *Optimally, feedback should not be given in front of peers*—especially if it is negative feedback. Even positive feedback given in front of peers may unintentionally foster competition or embarrass the individual. Many of us remember the pain of a lesson taught through humiliation during rounds in front of our peers or in morbidity and mortality rounds.

11. *Use the "sandwich technique."* This is a method of giving negative feedback in which concerns are "sandwiched" between positive feedback statements. An example of this regarding a resident's presentation of a case in a mock boards scenario would be: "The rate of your presentation was just right—it took up most of the 30 minutes. However, you forgot to address the patient's cognitive function in your mental status examination. Still, your formulation was complete, giving the biological, psychological, and sociocultural precipitants, predisposition, prognostic factors, patterns and treatment plan." This approach may make it easier to hear concerns without becoming defensive. It can backfire, however, if it sugarcoats or obscures an important piece of negative feedback, so it is crucial to pay attention to whether the learner has heard the meaning of the remarks.

12. *Communicate your appreciation.* Simply saying "thanks" is another form of feedback that communicates that one is aware of the other's effort and thankful for his or her contribution. Just this simple acknowledgement can encourage learning and development.

## SMART STRATEGIES

- Set expectations and objectives ahead of time and meet regularly.
- Begin by having students do a self-assessment.
- Measure objectively and be specific.
- Minimize defensiveness (use the "Columbo" approach).
- Attend to nonverbal communication.
- Give positive feedback prior to negative feedback (use the "sandwich" technique).
- Give timely feedback.
- Give feedback face to face or in writing if possible.
- Cite examples of behavior or performance that elicited the feedback.
- Give feedback one on one whenever possible.
- Catch people doing things right; look for opportunities to give positive feedback.
- Say "thank you."

## QUESTIONS TO DISCUSS WITH A MENTOR OR COLLEAGUE

1. Can you think of the last time you gave positive feedback?
2. Could you please give me positive and negative feedback?
3. What was the most memorable feedback you ever received, and why do you think it was memorable?
4. Have you ever given feedback you regretted giving? What was it you regretted?

## REFERENCES

Ende J: Feedback in clinical medical education. JAMA 250:777–781, 1983

Schum TR, Krippendorf RL, Biernat KA: Simple feedback notes enhance specificity of feedback to learners. Ambulatory Pediatrics 3:9–11, 2003

Whitman N, Weiss E, Lutz L: The Chief Resident as Manager, 2nd Edition. Salt Lake City, UT, Educational Dimensions, 1993, pp 79–87

## ADDITIONAL RESOURCES

Covey SR: The 7 Habits of Highly Effective People: Powerful Lessons in Personal Change. New York, Simon and Schuster, 1989

Nelson B: You Get What You Reward [Workforce Performance Web site]. June 1997. Available at: http://www.opm.gov/perform/articles/090.htm. Accessed February 13, 2005.

Stone D, Patton B, Heen S: Difficult Conversations: How to Discuss What Matters Most. New York, Penguin Books, 2000

Swinton L: Top 7 Tips on How to Give Positive Feedback [Top 7 Business Web site]. Available at: http://top7business.com/?top-7-tips-on-how-to-give-positive-feedback. Accessed February 13, 2005.

# CHAPTER 15

# Teaching and Helping Others to Learn

Malathi Srinivasan, M.D.

Donald M. Hilty, M.D.

Be the change you want to see in the world.

*Gandhi*

Physicians participate in educational endeavors for many reasons. They may want to be agents of change or enjoy interactions with learners. They may wish to expand the perspectives of learners, model desired behaviors, impart hard-won kernels of information, or have an impact on society through the dissemination of knowledge. Although they are content experts, few physicians have had formal training in teaching methods. Faculty are often unaware of their own teaching styles, choosing their teaching methods based on experiences in their own training (Leamon et al. 2002).

Teaching and learning do not occur in a vacuum. Therefore, this chapter reviews the factors that come to bear on teaching and learning, in a broad context, as well as ideas to prepare for and succeed with each teaching encounter.

## THE CONTEXT OF TEACHING AND LEARNING

Teaching is only one of several responsibilities of early career faculty members, and it occurs in a complex social network of a hospital or school of medicine. With an increasing number physicians choosing teaching as their career in medicine, it is gaining increased importance.

With institutional finances limited, deans, department chairs, or program directors—who may not teach, but who control the learning environment and culture—hire educators, select learners, create learning tools, and finance learning. Thus, a single educator is unlikely to have individual control over the global learning environment.

Faculty members may not think about the critical difference between teaching and learning. *Teaching* is the process of imparting information, in which the faculty member is usually the content expert or facilitator. *Learning* is the process of assimilating that information and should be the goal of any educational endeavor. In this case, learners may be medical students, residents, practicing physicians, academic colleagues, patients, legislators, or even private or public sector groups.

Our current educational system in academic medicine focuses on the process of teaching, using such metrics as the number of lecture hours, types of curriculum developed, weeks on inpatient or consult wards, and number of attending rounds. Our system does not routinely attend to the most critical component of instruction: did the learner learn during the educational encounter?

Therefore, to be effective promoters of learning, faculty members need new skill sets and must ask themselves strategic questions (Table 15–1). First, what are the common teaching and learning styles? Second, what methods will be used to engage learners? Third, what measures will evaluate success in teaching—did the learner learn? How will your learners know that they have learned?

The National Research Council is the national educational academy for the United States, with an advisory role to Congress and the public like those of the Institute of Medicine and the National Academy of Science. The National Research Council provides an resource on learning in their book *How People Learn*, which reviews the scientific basis of learning and memory, with an emphasis on learner predisposition, knowledge and skill acquisition, and approaches to learning and teaching (National Research Council 2000).

## FAMILIARITY WITH TEACHING AND LEARNING STYLES

As an educator, you should be familiar with some items of the commonly shared lexicon, and accompanying skill set, of teaching and learning styles. There are many learning theories, which inform different approaches to education. Although it may seem that these theories

**TABLE 15–1.** Strategic considerations in preparing for teaching and promoting learning

**Educator**

*Your motivation*

Why have you agreed to participate in this teaching encounter?

Part of your job description

Favor to a colleague

It's an important topic

In your area of expertise

You like the learner(s)

Want to learn about the topic

What are your competing responsibilities?

Other classes and courses

Patient care

Research

Administrative work

Professional meetings

Personal life

*Your skill sets*

What teaching strategies do you prefer to use?

What little-used teaching strategies could help you be effective?

What new skills do you need?

*You and your learners*

What do you know about the learner or group of learners?

What are your learners' needs?

How will you handle mixed learner groups (more and less advanced, both in the same setting?)

How will you promote active learning in all learner groups?

*Your goals*

What are you trying to accomplish (e.g., knowledge, skills, attitudes, other)?

How will you impart your goals to the learner?

*Your preparation*

How much encounter time do you have?

Do you have enough time to meet your goals?

Have you mobilized the appropriate resources to be effective?

Have you scheduled time to prepare to teach or learn?

Are you up to date for this content area?

What educational resources do you need?

What have other educators done that has been effective or ineffective?

---

**TABLE 15–1.**    Strategic considerations in preparing for teaching and promoting learning *(continued)*

---

What past barriers have influenced this educational encounter?

Can you use or modify pre-prepared material for lecture and discussion?

Which techniques are best suited to your goals?

*Your evaluation*

How will you evaluate your learner's success?

How will you evaluate your own success?

**Learner**

*Administrative*

What administrative resources do you have?

Who will schedule rooms and meetings? Who will page or contact learners?

Who will follow up with learners, take notes, and photocopy material?

Who can learners contact to reach you (given your hectic schedule)?

*Setting*

What is your preferred setting for your educational encounter: clinic, workroom, bedside, classroom, your office?

Will you mix learning environments?

Do you have access to critical resources or people who can help you?

How will you and your learners handle interruptions to the teaching encounter (cell phone, pagers, nurses, secretaries, patients)?

*Culture*

What are the cultural norms for your academic institution?

Are you aware of your biases towards institutional culture (the culture of your training program vs. your current institution)?

What are the unspoken rules of the institution that impact teaching?

Do learners expect you to give them assignments?

How do learners react to more directive interactions? Less directive interactions?

---

are mutually exclusive, educators commonly draw from several theories during their teaching sessions. An excellent Web resource from the United Kingdom that reviews these learning theories is James Atherton's "doceo" Web site http://www.learningandteaching.info/learning. Major learning theories include the following:

- Behavioral learning theory (Skinner, Thorndike, Watson): Learning occurs through behavioral change in the learner and is improved by reinforcement.

- Cognitive learning theory (Piaget, Kohler, Koffka): Learning is manifested by changes in the learner's internal state of development, through progressive addition of new knowledge. Educators start "where the learner is," probe understanding, use gestalt theories, cognitive dissonance, and assimilation strategies, and help learners synthesize and adapt new information.
- Constructivist learning theory (Dewey, Piaget, Bruner): Based on cognitive learning theory. Examines how learners construct their knowledge of the world around them. Learning is a joint endeavor between learners and teachers, with learners as the "makers of meanings."
- Social learning theory (Vygotsky, Bruner): Learning occurs best in simulations or in actual practice. Learners practice and become socialized into behavioral roles and the culture of the profession through role modeling.
- Inspirational learning theory (Palmer 1998): Learning occurs as educators inspire learners with passion, integrity, authenticity, connectedness, and caring.

Learning theories and teaching approaches were the subject of Pratt and Collins's work, culminating in their *Five Perspectives on Teaching in Adult and Higher Education* (Pratt et al. 1998), for which they had interviewed more than 250 award-winning educators from multiple disciplines about their interactions with learners. Five major perspectives emerged from their work (merged with the social reform perspective of Kember [1997], as articulated in Table 15–2). In this model, the educators' perspectives vary by their predominant desires to influence the interaction between themselves, their learners, and the environment in which learning occurs. Educators usually have one or two perspectives that are dominant. Pratt and Collins's Teaching Perspectives Inventory has been taken by more than 22,000 educators and is available free of charge at http://www.teachingperspectives.com.

Kolb described learner-centered styles in his 1984 work *Experiential Learning,* building on several existing models and drawing mainly from cognitive learning theory. Lewin's "cycle of adult learning" (Lewin 1948) is used to outline a sequence of four steps used to achieve understanding (Figure 15–1); the learner may enter the cycle at any time. Using this cycle, Honey and Mumford (1982) described four types of dominant learning styles: activist, reflector, theorist, and pragmatist. Kolb's work on "experiential learning" drew these theories together in innovative ways. He developed an instrument to measure the propensity of learners to use one

**TABLE 15–2.** Five teaching perspectives

| Perspective | Beliefs | Intentions | Actions | Common setting |
|---|---|---|---|---|
| **Transmission** | Effective teaching requires a substantial commitment to the content or subject matter. (*focus: educator ↔ content*) | Teachers' primary responsibilities are to represent the content accurately and efficiently. Learners' responsibilities are to learn content in its authorized or legitimate forms. | Good teachers take learners systematically through tasks leading to content mastery. They provide objectives, efficiently use class time, clarify misunderstandings, answer questions, provide timely feedback, summarize, and develop objective means of assessing learning. | Lecture. |

**TABLE 15–2.**   Five teaching perspectives *(continued)*

| Perspective | Beliefs | Intentions | Actions | Common setting |
|---|---|---|---|---|
| **Apprenticeship** *(social learning theory)* | Effective teaching is a process of socializing students into new behavioral norms and ways of working. *(focus: educator ↔ content)* | Teachers must reveal the inner workings of skilled performance. Learning occurs in the context of practice, and the learners are socialized in acceptable normative behaviors. Learning is translated into accessible language and a set of tasks, from simple to complex, allowing for different points of entry. | Good teachers are highly skilled practitioners of what they teach. They know what their learners can do on their own and where they need guidance and direction; they engage learners within their "zone of development." As learners become more competent, the teacher offers less direction and gives more responsibility. For instance, modeling behaviors in the apprenticeship model could include communication/counseling/interpersonal skills or physical skills such as laparotomy. | Skills development in any setting: clinic, inpatient ward, operating room. |

**TABLE 15–2.**   Five teaching perspectives *(continued)*

| Perspective | Beliefs | Intentions | Actions | Common setting |
|---|---|---|---|---|
| **Developmental** *(cognitive theory)* | Effective teaching must be planned and conducted from the learner's point of view, exploring the learner's a priori understanding. *(focus: learner ↔ content)* | Teachers must understand how their learners think and reason about the content—probing of learner knowledge. The primary goal is to help learners develop increasingly complex and sophisticated cognitive structures for comprehending the content. | Good teachers adapt their teaching to learners' levels of understanding and ways of thinking. Changing knowledge structure and facilitating new forms of reasoning can be accomplished through 1) questioning, to move learners from simple to more complex thought, and 2) bridging knowledge with meaningful examples. | Internal medicine or psychiatry team rounds. |

**TABLE 15–2.** Five teaching perspectives *(continued)*

| Perspective | Beliefs | Intentions | Actions | Common setting |
|---|---|---|---|---|
| Nurturing | Effective teaching assumes that long-term, hard, and persistent efforts toward achievement come from the heart of the learner, not just their intellect. *(focus: educator ↔ learner)* | People become motivated and productive learners when working on issues or problems without fear. Learners are nurtured in knowing that 1) they can succeed at learning if they try; 2) achievement is a product of their own effort and ability, rather than the benevolence of a teacher; and 3) learning efforts will be supported by others. | Good teachers care about their students and understand that some have histories of failure resulting in lowered self-confidence. However they make no excuses for learners. Rather, they encourage their efforts while challenging students to do their best by promoting a climate of caring and trust, with challenging but achievable goals and support. | Any setting in which small group or individual interactions can occur. |

**TABLE 15–2.** Five teaching perspectives *(continued)*

| Perspective | Beliefs | Intentions | Actions | Common setting |
|---|---|---|---|---|
| **Social reform** | Effective teaching seeks to change society in substantive ways. *(focus: learner ↔ context)* | From the social reform point of view, the object of teaching is the collective rather than the individual. | Good teachers awaken students to values and ideologies that are embedded in texts and common practices within their disciplines. Good teachers challenge the status quo and encourage students to consider how learners are positioned. Texts are interrogated for what is (or not) said and included and who is (or is not) represented from the dominant discourse. | Any setting. |

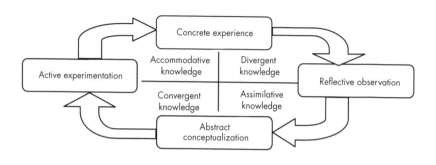

**FIGURE 15–1.** Kolb's experiential learning, with Lewin's cycle/spiral of active learning.
*Source.* Adapted from Kolb 1984.

of these four learning styles and the types of knowledge that each group may generate or utilize (Figure 15–1). He also classified different professions as preferentially falling within these four quadrants of knowledge. For a nominal charge, you can complete the copyrighted Learning Styles Inventory (http://www.learningfromexperience.com) and obtain further information about these knowledge types.

## DEFINING THE EDUCATIONAL ENCOUNTER

Before choosing a teaching method or location, an educator must first ask, "What do I want to accomplish?" Areas for learner improvement might include

- Cognitive knowledge about topic
- Skills acquisition (procedural, communication, leadership)
- Changes in attitude or beliefs
- Improved self-efficacy
- Development of beneficial self-learning strategies
- Development of professional habits and interaction skills

You must understand where your particular topic falls within the overall learning schema for this set of learners. This will allow you to maximize the impact of your time with the learners and be justly rewarded (Table 15–3).

What teaching method is best for your purposes? Is there more than one? The literature abounds with multiple teaching methods: problem-

---

**TABLE 15–3.**     Questions about teaching for the dean, department chair, or program director

---

**Curricular continuity**

Where have similar skills and information been taught in the curriculum?

Has this topic been taught? Do you have access to material the previous instructor used? To the instructor?

Where will your topic fall in the curricular schema?

Can you overtly link or reference prior classes? ("*As Dr. Lee said last week during…*")

Can the skills and information you teach be reinforced in other portions of the curriculum?

**Learner a priori knowledge**

What are learners likely to know already?

Have they practiced what they know?

Are learners ready to learn or are there cultural or institutional barriers that might inhibit them?

**Educator preparation**

How much time will encounters with learners take to prepare and evaluate?

If the time is significant, will this count toward your promotion, salary, or other incentive?

If the time is significant, can other things be taken off your plate?

How will course evaluations be used in your promotion or career?

Do you need to ask for resources that will contribute to curricular success?

---

based learning, lecture formats, bedside teaching, Socratic dialogue, communication skills workshops, videotape reviews, standardized patient interviews, observed encounters, independent learning modules, and others. The size of the group coupled with the educational goals often determine the methods used to teach (Tables 15–4 and 15–5). Each method has advantages and disadvantages. While information dissemination is easy to accomplish in a large group setting, it is difficult to assess an individual's pace of learning or his or her skills acquisition (Tables 15–6 and 15–7). Similarly, a small group setting is resource-intensive but is also conducive to facilitated, engaging interactions (see Chapter 16 in this volume).

## DEFINING SUCCESS

What constitutes success in your curriculum or educational interaction? Your educational goals should be important, discrete, and achievable

**TABLE 15–4.** Larger and medium-sized groups

| Number of learners | Goal | Setting | Potential instructional method |
|---|---|---|---|
| >30 (large) and 12–30 (medium) | Acquire information | Classroom | • Syllabus or preassigned reading<br>• Lectures |
| | | Self-study | • Computer modules<br>• Paper modules<br>• Self-assessment with formative and summative testing<br>• Creation of Web-based learning communities |
| | Develop skills | Classroom | • Break-out sessions within large group<br>• Field trips to see patients or skill centers<br>• Demonstration of techniques by experts<br>• Role-playing and feedback with individual volunteers |
| | Assess attitude | Classroom | • Interactive question and answer response systems<br>• Preclass surveys (Web-based or paper) |
| | | Informal settings | • Informal discussion and role modeling<br>• Elicitation of biases and preconceptions |
| | Assess knowledge | Classroom | • Interactive question and answer response systems<br>• Preclass surveys (Web-based or paper)<br>• Reflective moments: learners asked to self-assess |
| | Assess skills | Classroom | • Baseline and interval assessment in break-out sessions<br>• Self-assessment with interactive question and answer systems |

*Note.* The challenge of large group settings is addressing heterogeneity in learner knowledge and effectively engaging all learners in the topic. Techniques to increase interaction and interval assessment are used to meet different educational goals. The curriculum and goals must be extremely clear and must focus on clarity of presentation.

**TABLE 15–5.** Small and very small groups

| Number of learners | Goal | Setting | Potential instructional method |
|---|---|---|---|
| 3–12 (small) | Acquire knowledge | Classroom or bedside | • Learner presentation, with question and answer period<br>• Socratic dialogue, exploring learner knowledge |
| | Develop skills | Classroom or conference room | • Preassigned reading and assignments<br>• Educator-directed group discussion<br>  •Case-based learning<br>• Learner-directed group discussion<br>  •Problem-based learning<br>• Learner presentation, with question and answer period |
| | | Bedside | • Educator demonstration at bedside<br>• Direct observation of learners at bedside<br>• Videotaping of patient–learner interactions |
| | | Conference | • Videotape review<br>• Review of patient–learner interactions with group<br>  • Open discussion<br>  • Standardized feedback methodology |
| | | Standardized patients | • Standardized patient–learner interactions with time out for discussion and "re-try" of techniques<br>• Standardized patient–learner interaction for formative evaluation |
| | Attitude | All settings | • Discussion of barriers and facilitators to behaviors |
| | | Informal settings | • Informal discussion and role modeling |

**TABLE 15–5.** Small and very small groups *(continued)*

| Number of learners | Goal | Setting | Potential instructional method |
|---|---|---|---|
| 1–2 (very small) | Acquire knowledge | Classroom or bedside | • Learner presentation, with question and answer period<br>• Socratic dialogue, exploring learner knowledge<br>• Testing and individual answer review |
| | Develop skills | Classroom | • Review of patient–learner interactions (or standardized patient–learner interactions) in group (low level of personal feedback) |
| | | Bedside | • Observation of patient–learner interaction (live or videotaped) |
| | Attitude | All settings | • Mentorship, informal and formal<br>• Discussion of barriers and facilitators to behaviors |

*Note.* In small groups, facilitated interactions by educators are possible, with individual attention to the learner's phase of learning. Small groups are found in all academic settings. This method of teaching is extremely resource intensive. Unless faculty training is conducted appropriately, faculty evaluation of learners may be extremely subjective and result in large reporting biases.

**TABLE 15–6.** Example analysis of instructional method: lectures

| | |
|---|---|
| Method | • Lecture format: four 1-hour talks on schizophrenia |
| Dominant learning theory | • Constructivism or cognitive |
| Dominant teaching perspective | • Transmission |
| Advantages | • Conveys large amounts of material in a time-efficient manner |
| | • Allows a demonstration of skills (e.g., how to interview a patient). |
| | • Presents and discusses concepts and integrates information |
| | • Conducts question and answer sessions with time-strapped experts. |
| | • Necessary faculty training may be minimal, since many are experienced. |
| | • Course and lecture evaluations based on understandable surveys and tests. |
| Disadvantages | • No in-depth assessment of learner's knowledge. |
| | • Cannot ascertain if learners are learning. |
| | • Challenging to tailor information to different learner levels. |
| | • Tendency to present too much information in a session. |
| | • Topic should be evaluated in light of adjacent teaching sessions (e.g., are there four lectures in a row on one morning?). |
| | • Without a clear understanding of where a topic fits into the learner's curriculum, faculty may provide unclear, redundant, or conflicting information. |

**TABLE 15–6.** Example analysis of instructional method: lectures *(continued)*

| Methods to overcome disadvantages | **Before the lecture:** |
|---|---|
| | • Negotiate and finalize learning objectives, as well as time and resources needed. |
| | • Narrow objectives and content to be conveyed; less is more. |
| | • Assess learners' knowledge, skills, and attitudes with surveys. |
| | • Provide homework or precourse assignments that facilitate information integration. |
| | • Ask colleague to observe lecture and give you pointers on improvement. |
| | **During the lecture:** |
| | • Convey expectations and objectives to learners at beginning of lecture. |
| | • Convey relevancy with vibrant useful examples ("Last week in clinic…"). |
| | • Address common misconceptions ("How many of you think that…?"). |
| | • Use interactive teaching elements to engage learners: |
| |    • Case presentation and discussion |
| |    • Audience response systems |
| |    • In-class questions about content |
| |    • Break-out sessions, task development, and group leaders report back |
| |    • Stop lecture and solicit understanding or questions from learners |
| |    • Bring in live discussants, patients, policy advocates, visiting experts |
| | • Break-out sessions may take 30 minutes or more; cut into time and must narrow objectives. |
| | • Challenge learners to think in class with provocative statements; ask for responses. |
| | **After the lecture:** |
| | • Ask for feedback from learners at the end of lecture. |
| | • Develop summative test items that assess key points from your lecture. |
| | • Self-critique: what was done well and what could have been done better? |

**TABLE 15–6.**   Example analysis of instructional method: lectures *(continued)*

| Resources needed | |
|---|---|
| | • Review of national standards and competency development standards. |
| | • Brief review of learners' curriculum (where does your lecture fall in their courses?). |
| | • Obtain presentation material: |
| |     • Images from national databases (i.e., The Complete Human, etc.) |
| |     • Clinical cases from educator databanks |
| |     • Prior lectures from colleagues and past years; don't reinvent |
| | • Administrative support to copy, disseminate, collect, and score material. |
| | • Carve out adequate time to prepare lecture and review outcomes. |
| | • Audiovisual support where necessary. |
| | • Find colleague to help offer critique. |

---

**TABLE 15-7.** Tips for a lecture setting

---

**Focusing your presentation**

- Identify your learning objectives and key points. Discuss them with a colleague.
- Narrow your learning objectives— focus on key concepts, and flesh out concepts with important facts that will affect their practice.
- Imagine yourself in the learner's shoes—what would bore you?
- Practice. You need to be prepared. What makes you nervous?

**Timing your presentation**

*A common format for an hour-long topic review is…*

- Present case illustration, story, or starter question as introduction (3 minutes)
- Ask a few questions: "By show of hands, how many of your are familiar with…? How many of you take care of…"
- Discuss format of the hour (1 minute)
- Discuss epidemiology and importance of topic (2 minutes; mention only 3–5 points)
- Give quick pathophysiology review (3 minutes; use an animated illustration to build your physiology)
- Discuss state of the art in this topic (15–20 minutes; pick 3–6 topics and create just one major slide on each)
- Stop the lecture and ask for questions at some point during the lecture; think of other interactive ideas (5 minutes)
- Discuss implications of these advances for practice, policy, patients (3 minutes)
- Summarize (2 minutes)
- Question slide, with gratuitous picture of your family or your dog
- Allow discussion (10–15 minutes)

**Using PowerPoint or slides**

- These should be learning aids, not teaching crutches. You need to be prepared. Less is more.
- Don't read off your slides. Use them to help discuss your topic, not substitute for a discussion. Again, you need to be prepared.
- Maximum limit: 6 lines per slide. No more than 8–10 words per line. No more than 20 words for an hour talk.
- Illustrations and graphs: help your learner orient to the slide. "This chart shows you the effectiveness of drug X in middle aged schizophrenic patients. The X-axis represents….and the Y-axis represents….You can see that the two lines converge…."

---

for the learner. They should be linked to specific competency domains important to your program and should have demonstrable outcomes (Table 15–8). Although it may seem like a cumbersome exercise, the process of identifying the competency domain, specifying discrete learning objectives, and defining achievable goals for each learning objective allows the educator to understand what is achievable in an educational setting. It also helps you, the educator, to understand what is achievable, given your resources. Outcome measurements may need to be spread longitudinally, in multiple courses or rotations, or tested in collaboration with other institutions.

We would encourage medical educators to peruse the Web site http://www.acgme.org and review some current definitions of physician competency by specialty. Many tools are emerging for skills assessment, including standardized patient interactions and checklists, roleplaying exercises, and "shelf exams" for tests of knowledge. Depending on your resources and desired impact, you may decide to assess outcomes at the learner, curricular, patient, system, or societal level.

## SMART STRATEGIES

- Be aware of the learner, course, department, school, hospital, and health system factors that come to bear on your teaching.
- Learn about your teaching style by taking a teaching inventory.
- Learn about, and draw from, the learning styles of your trainees and other faculty.
- Be specific with your teaching goals, methods, and targeted outcomes, and choose a tool for assessment that fits your learning environment, goal, and time frame.
- Take a teaching scholars seminar, perhaps with others in psychiatry or medicine, to develop your skills.
- Attend a meeting of a national organization that is focused on teaching, such as the Association for Academic Psychiatry (http://www.academicpsychiatry.org), the Society of Teachers in Family Medicine (http://www.stfm.org), the American Association of Medical Colleges (http://www.aamc.org) and that organization's Research in Medical Education section (http://www.aamc.org/members/gea/rimesection/start.htm), the Accreditation Council for Graduate Medical Education educators' meetings (http://www.acgme.org, meetings and workshops tab), and the Society for General Internal Medicine (http://www.sgim.org).

**TABLE 15–8.** Development of outcomes tracking with learning objectives and goals

| Domain of interest | Outcome area | Assessment tools |
|---|---|---|
| **Individual learning objectives** | | |
| Goal 1 | Improved attitude: assess attitudes, biases, knowledge of schizophrenia, and issues in conducting family meetings with patients with schizophrenia. | • Pre-post survey of attitudes of residents.<br>• Solicitation of biases and preconceptions about disease.<br>• Discussion in group settings. |
| Goal 2 | Improved knowledge: assess knowledge and application of knowledge in family conference. | • Tests of cognitive knowledge—set predetermined standard of achievement. Ensure that knowledge tests address key learning objectives.<br>• Feedback about how knowledge was used in clinical settings. |

*(continued)*

**TABLE 15–8.** Development of outcomes tracking with learning objectives and goals *(continued)*

| Domain of interest | Outcome area | Assessment tools |
|---|---|---|
| | Improved skills: assess appropriate use of communication styles during family conference. | • Patient and family survey. Did they…<br>   • Feel understood?<br>   • Have questions answered at appropriate level?<br>   • Feel that their issues were resolved at end?<br>   • Have a manageable follow-up plan?<br>• Faculty feedback about resident performance<br>   • Skillful utilization of communication styles?<br>   • Set an open environment?<br>   • Address major issues in the encounter?<br>• Resident self-assessment of performance |
| | Improved habits: assess sustained habits of resident during future encounters. | • Resident self-report<br>• Longitudinal observation by faculty<br>• Videotape review with faculty<br>• Standardized patient interviews<br>• Chart audits |

**TABLE 15–8.** Development of outcomes tracking with learning objectives and goals *(continued)*

| Domain of interest | Outcome area | Assessment tools |
|---|---|---|
| Curricular outcomes | Learner satisfaction.<br>Faculty satisfaction.<br>Learner performance outcomes.<br>Patient outcomes. | • Tailored survey of relevant groups<br>• Assessment of aggregate learner outcomes |
| Specific outcomes[a]<br>Example: Goal 3 | Tailor communication style of learner during family conference.<br>1. Be able to verbalize major communication styles and techniques: shared decision-making, nondirective counseling, directive counseling, open- and closed-ended approaches, setting a welcoming environment, etc.<br>2. Be able to role-play common scenarios: "What will you do if the family becomes irritated with the patient during the encounter and begins to verbally fight with each other?" | |

*(continued)*

**TABLE 15–8.**  Development of outcomes tracking with learning objectives and goals *(continued)*

| Domain of interest | Outcome area | Assessment tools |
|---|---|---|
| | 3. Demonstrate flexibility during the family encounter, and switch from style to style. | |
| | 4. Consciously use different communication techniques in the encounter. | |
| | 5. Discuss the techniques they use, and *why*, after the encounter in debriefing session. | |

[a]Specific outcomes and assessment tools increase in specificity, from the general outcomes of interest for learning objectives to very specific outcomes that can be assessed for goals. Note that the goals listed can be concretely defined and should, whenever possible, be low inference. Also note that the goals are written for "competent practice"—not for early or late beginners, nor for experts or masters of their field. Curricular and system outcomes should also be assessed when possible.

## QUESTIONS TO DISCUSS WITH A MENTOR OR COLLEAGUE

1. How do I assess my teaching skills, and what do I need to do to improve?
2. What resources do the department, school, hospital, and health system have in place that I can access (e.g., teaching resource center, seminar series, mentoring)?
3. What national organizations facilitate faculty development in education, and which one suits my personal goals?

## REFERENCES

Honey P, Mumford A: Manual of Learning Styles. London, Peter Honey Publications, 1982

Kolb DA: Experiential Learning: Experience as the Source of Learning and Development. Englewood Cliffs, NJ, Prentice-Hall, 1984

Leamon MH, Cox PD, Servis M: Educational perspectives: a discussion of teaching among colleagues. Acad Psychiatry 26:61–69, 2002

National Research Council: How People Learn: Brain, Mind, Experience and School. Washington, DC, National Academy Press, 2000

Palmer PJ: The Courage to Teach: Exploring the Inner Landscape of a Teacher's Life. San Francisco, CA, Jossey-Bass, 1998

Pratt DD, Collins J, associates: Five Perspectives on Teaching in Adult and Higher Education. Malabar, FL, Krieger, 1998

## ADDITIONAL RESOURCES

Accreditation Council for Continuing Medical Education:
http://www.accme.org
American Board of Medical Specialties: http://www.abms.org
Definitions of competency: http://www.acgme.org
James Atherton's doceo site: http://www.learningandteaching.info
Learning styles inventory: http://www.learningfromexperience.com
Teaching perspectives used by teachers:
http://www.teachingperspectives .com

# CHAPTER 16

# Teaching in
# Small Group Settings

Hendry Ton, M.D.

Donald M. Hilty, M.D.

Michael S. Wilkes, M.D.

Small groups can be an effective tool for learning at all levels of medical education. Small group teaching can be particularly well suited for psychiatrists, who have training in group therapy and are therefore effective at evaluating and facilitating group processes. This teaching modality has been gaining popularity since 1969, when McMaster University in Ontario established North America's first problem-based learning curriculum, which relies extensively on small groups (Donner and Bickley 1993). Medical educators are now frequently asked to lead small groups.

The small group has a number of advantages and disadvantages compared with traditional didactic teaching (Table 16–1). In general, small groups encourage students to be more active learners and to develop interpersonal skills. Although there are some disadvantages, the educational benefits of small groups generally outweigh these largely logistical limitations. This chapter focuses on types of small group formats, effective use of groups in education, and evaluation of small group teaching. We will also attempt to point out differences between small groups that meet only a few times (e.g., one to four sessions) and more longitudinal small groups (e.g., those that meet over the course of an academic year).

**TABLE 16–1.**   Pros and cons of small group teaching

| Pros | Cons |
|------|------|
| • Promotes more lasting and meaningful learning | • Requires more time per learning issue |
| • Promotes problem solving and critical thinking | • Requires learner preparation and active participation |
| • Develops learning as a skill | • Requires greater faculty-to-learner ratio |
| • Improves teaching skills of group members | • May have more variability in faculty quality |
| • Improves interpersonal and teamwork skills | • May be more costly to implement |
| • Can provide a support structure among students | • May be more complex to coordinate |

## LEARNING OBJECTIVES

In preparation for small group teaching, it is important to delineate the learning objectives for learners *and* teachers in order to select the teaching method that optimizes the chances of delivering planned outcomes. Potential objectives for learners may include improving knowledge and skills (clinical, teaching, interpersonal, or collaborative skills), developing attitudes, and promoting support. For teachers, objectives may similarly include improving knowledge and skills (clinical, teaching, and mentoring skills), developing attitudes, and facilitating peer support. As outlined earlier, improving knowledge may be better accomplished in other formats (e.g., lecture), particularly if a large quantity is to be dispensed. On the other hand, skills (e.g., how to start an interview, how to give bad news) and attitudes may be better taught in a small group, which may reduce the anxiety of participants, allow learners to observe and give feedback to each other, and allow for role modeling among peers. Notably, many goals can be accomplished in short-term group sessions, but attainments like socialization and professional attitudes and skills may require a long-term, integrated program (see also Chapter 17).

## SMALL GROUP FORMATS

There are many formats for small group teaching. Two in common use for small groups are *case-based* and *problem-based* formats. In the case-based approach, learners work through realistic clinical cases—the case itself provides structure for discussing the lesson issues. Case-based sessions may be easier for faculty to prepare because many of the learning issues can be written into the case beforehand. Cases also add relevance to learning issues for medical students and faculty, thereby improving the motivation to learn. In problem-based learning, students are given a problem that typically reflects a real world issue. They then collectively work to define the problem, identify what information is needed, and discuss solutions. Although participation is essential for both formats, active learning and teamwork skills are stressed to a greater degree in problem-based learning formats. The relative lack of structure may pose a challenge to the facilitator and learners alike, and may obscure the relevance of the session. Small groups may incorporate elements of both formats, as they are not mutually exclusive.

## SUPPLEMENTAL TEACHING TOOLS

Use of supplemental teaching tools can enhance learning in small groups; learners need to have adequate resources to work through learning topics. However, it is important to align these supplements appropriately to the learning objectives of the small group session to enhance rather than detract from the learning process.

### Audiovisual Aids

Computer-based presentations work well for teacher-oriented groups but may impede learner-directed groups. However, if properly used, audiovisual aids can add structure to a small group session and appeal to various sensory modalities. An overhead projector, for example, places the teacher with the learners and if used correctly, can incorporate learners' views (e.g., with teaching points and questions to generate a list). Multimedia videos of patient interactions stimulate discussion more effectively than paper cases. Facilitators should be aware, however, that overuse of audiovisual aids may actually impede group process and put students in a more passive role.

### Standardized Patients

Standardized patients (SPs), individuals who play the role of a patient in physician training, can be a particularly useful teaching aid for courses emphasizing interviews. They enable learners to test strategies for addressing challenging interactions with patients—and to get timely feedback from facilitators and peers about these strategies. Other students in the group also benefit from observing and discussing the interviews. Care should be taken when facilitating feedback, because students may feel put on the spot and vulnerable to criticism from the group. Students may also feel that the interview is contrived if the SPs are poorly trained. Some strategies to improve the quality of SPs include recruiting actors or those with acting skills and trainers who have experience preparing the SPs.

## Assigned Readings

Adequate preparation by students is essential for successful groups. Assigned readings can help ensure that the group has enough knowledge about the topics to initiate discussion for active learning. Essential articles should be given to all members of the group, whereas supplemental readings can be assigned to specific members of the group, who can then teach other members.

## Lectures

Similar to assigned readings, lectures can be used to help prepare students for their small group discussion. A lecture has advantages over assigned readings in that it requires less student preparation time (which is often an issue for trainees), is more interactive, and typically uses several different sensory modalities for learning. Lectures can also be tailored to specifically fit the learning objectives, whereas finding an article to do this may be challenging.

Lecturing in small groups is generally discouraged because it puts students in the passive role and impedes the small group process. However, facilitators can sparingly interject knowledge to facilitate discussion when students are at an impasse and need a base of knowledge to jump-start the discussion. Because one of the most significant problems in small group teaching is lecturing by facilitators, this modality should be used very sparingly.

## COMPOSITION AND STRUCTURE

Successful group teaching requires a context that is conducive to learning. Ideally, small groups should consist of 6 to 10 individuals. Diversity of gender, backgrounds, interests, and perspectives can also promote rich exploration of the learning topics. However, separating individuals with preestablished conflicts may help maximize the potential for group cohesion. Groups should be conducted in rooms that are designed to fit their size; rooms that are too large, in particular, may impede the development of safety and intimacy in the group. Members of the group sit so that they can easily see each other, which typically entails sitting in as close to a circular format as possible. There are also advantages to co-facilitators sitting apart from each other: this conveys the importance of group members taking ownership of the process and enables the facilitators to cover more area collectively when visually monitoring the group process. Facilitators should also monitor the level of energy of the group and allow for breaks when fatigue sets in. This is especially important for long sessions. Role designation facilitates learning, with role options including scribes to write down key points, presenters of articles, timekeepers, interviewers, and others.

## GROUP LEADERSHIP

Effective leadership is essential for successful small group learning. Leaders must help to establish a positive and safe learning environment, facilitate group process, and help the group adhere to the learning objectives. Specific personal qualities, knowledge, and skills enable leaders to do this. Interestingly, group leaders vary: in short-term groups, leaders are generally faculty; in long-term groups, both faculty and learners take on the leadership role.

### Personal Attributes

Effective facilitators model attentiveness, supportiveness, and respect. This stance mitigates the concerns of many students about having the right answer and encourages students to take chances more often in the discussions. Facilitators who are honest about their own limitations also encourage honest self-assessment within the group and promote collaboration. It is important for facilitators to have and express enthusiasm for the learning process, because their energy level strongly influences the group's overall energy level. These attributes help the facilitator to establish a safe and stimulating context for learning.

### Knowledge

It is essential that facilitators adequately prepare for the small group session by becoming familiar with the learning topics. Being well prepared enables facilitators to assess the group's progress with regard to the learning objectives and to guide the direction of discussion to keep the group on track. It is also useful to have a sense of the group's initial and longitudinal

**TABLE 16–2.**   Normative stages of group development

| Stage | Facilitation challenges |
| --- | --- |
| 1. Defining and structuring procedures<br>• Initial concern for the nature of the course<br>• Dependence on authority in group | • High group dependence on facilitator<br>• Clarify tasks, explain procedures, prepare the group to work with one another<br>• Model behaviors |
| 2. Conforming to procedures and getting acquainted<br>• Group becomes familiar with and conforms to procedures and norms of group<br>• Facilitators necessary for direction<br>• Individuals do not yet feel personal commitment to group's goals | |
| 3. Recognizing mutuality and building trust<br>• Group recognizes interdependence and builds a sense of cooperation and trust<br>• Feeling of mutual support and collaboration | |

**TABLE 16–2.** Normative stages of group development *(continued)*

| Stage | Facilitation challenges |
| --- | --- |
| 4. Rebelling and differentiating<br>• Establish interpersonal boundaries and sense of autonomy that can lead to strong group identity<br>• Differences are asserted<br>• Resistance to previously accepted responsibilities<br>• Individuals may become more passive, less cooperative | • Don't tighten control or try to force conformity<br>• Reason and negotiate<br>• Mediate conflicts while helping to underpin autonomy and individuality<br>• Work toward members taking ownership of group and commitment to each other |
| 5. Ownership of group<br>• Group becomes "our group" rather than facilitator's group<br>• Internalizing group rules and procedures | |
| 6. Functioning maturely and productively<br>• Group functions optimally<br>• Able to operate in different modalities to achieve group goals and learning objectives<br>• Leadership is shared among members | • Facilitator serves as consultant and resource |
| 7. Termination<br>• Group comes to end, members move on | • Encourage discussion of termination<br>• Discuss members' overall experience of the group<br>• Discuss what has been accomplished and what still needs to be accomplished<br>• Facilitators and mentors give feedback |

*Source.* Adapted from Johnson DW, Johnson FP: "Research Into Group Behavior," in *Learning in Groups*. Edited by Jacques D. London, Kogan Page, 2000, pp 34–37; and from Johnson DW, Johnson FP: *Joining Together: Group Therapy and Group Skills*. Englewood Cliffs, NJ, Prentice Hall, 1990.

emotional state during the session because this invariably influences how the students will learn. This can be achieved effectively by asking students to check in at the beginning of the session (which would entail asking members how they have been since the last meeting of the group). Doing so enables facilitators to link discussion topics with the issues brought up during check-in when appropriate, thereby adding to the relevance of the learning process. Knowledge about normative group identity development over time can be useful for facilitators of long-term groups and can help put difficulties experienced in groups into context (Table 16–2). Short-term groups may go through some of these stages; long-term groups tend to go through all of them.

## Skills

Skillful facilitation of a group is arguably the most important thing that a leader can contribute. Paying close attention to group process is as important to small group teaching as it is to traditional group therapy. Table 16–3 summarizes guidelines for facilitating small groups. Table 16–4 highlights some common problems and suggested solutions. In addition to these solutions, problem behaviors can be brought up with the small group for members to collectively address. This method will not only improve the group's overall teamwork but may also work to improve members' ownership of the group process. Problems that continue to arise can also be addressed with the group member individually as well.

## EVALUATION, DOCUMENTATION, AND FEEDBACK

Evaluation of small group teaching is complex. For short-term groups (e.g., one to four sessions), teachers may get a gestalt sense of what happened, but this measure is often crude. In line with continuing medical education programs, it is advisable to generate three group objectives for a given hour for short-term groups and to generate both group and individual objectives for long-term groups. Time budgeted immediately after the group session should be used to debrief, evaluate performance, and set objectives for the next group, if applicable. If individual performances stand out in good or bad ways, those may be noted, too.

Documentation should be aligned with objectives, and a form can be used to organize the learning and evaluation process. More and more, teachers are being explicit about how the group and individual learners are evaluated (i.e., the assessment drives the curriculum) by giving learners the objectives and or measures by which they will be evaluated.

**TABLE 16–3.**    Guidelines for small group facilitation

| General principle | Tip |
|---|---|
| Allow adequate warm-up time. | • Ensure adequate check-in time and set goals for the session. |
| Allow students to struggle with difficult issues before stepping in. | • Allow time after posing a question.<br>• Do not answer it yourself, rephrase, or reframe.<br>• Count to 10 before speaking. |
| Facilitate multiple approaches to difficult situations. | • Encourage students to discuss their ideas to enrich the discussion and be active.<br>• If necessary, play devil's advocate. |
| Identify uninvolved learners and get them involved to diversify learning. | • Observe body language, and look for signs that they are looking for an opportunity to speak (i.e., restlessness, straightened posture, leaning forward).<br>• Encourage students to speak to each other, not just the facilitator. |
| Keep track of goals for session. | • Summarize and refocus group. |
| Enhance relevance. | • Provide brief personal anecdotes. |
| Establish and respect ground rules for open communication and safety. | • Include confidentiality if group has supportive role. |

Giving students an opportunity to evaluate the group as a whole, in addition to encouraging self-assessment and assessment of peers, further engages the student in the learning process and provides helpful insights for the faculty. Students should also evaluate the faculty. This can be done anonymously after the session. This feedback can improve facilitation in subsequent groups, inform the next session's goals when applicable, and document the faculty member's teaching and facilitation skills for academic promotion. Therefore, self-assessment by faculty members should be compared with learners' assessment of them.

Faculty should assess the small group overall as well as individual components (if there is more than one session). Faculty assessment of learners should be based on observable behaviors: interviewing skill, presenting skill, collaboration, attendance, and punctuality. Problem-solving skills, qualitative measures of attitudes, curiosity, and openness to new ideas may also be useful points of evaluation.

Feedback is necessary for all parties at the one-quarter, halfway, and

**TABLE 16–4.** Dealing with small group problems

| Problem issues | Suggestions |
| --- | --- |
| Side conversations | • Discuss ground rules.<br>• Ask group to refocus on the current discussion. |
| Dominant member | • Support and bring others into discussion.<br>• Assign roles for dominant members (e.g., time keeper). |
| Quiet member | • Invite member to join discussion, "What are your thoughts about this?"<br>• Look for nonverbal cues indicating that the member may be interested in saying something.<br>• Assign tasks (i.e., summarizing discussion). |
| Antagonistic member | • Assess why the member is hostile, "You seem unhappy with how things are going."<br>• Facilitate discussion of concerns about the small group format or process.<br>• Assess whether member feels supported or validated in group.<br>• Check in with overall group regarding safety.<br>• Rephrase member's comments in less confrontational ways. |
| Clown | • Ask member to make serious contributions to discussion.<br>• Reinforce or validate serious contributions member makes.<br>• Assign roles. |
| Ineffective facilitator | • Hold faculty development sessions for all facilitators to review session material and discuss facilitation issues.<br>• Meet individually with facilitator.<br>• Review videotapes with facilitator. |
| Tangential discussions | • Review objectives.<br>• Refocus discussion, "I'm wondering how this relates to our current issue."<br>• Make a process observation, "I noticed that we started out talking about topic A, and now we are talking about topic B. Is this where we want to go?" |

three-quarter point marks, as well as at the end (see Chapter 14). Even if the group meets only once or twice, a check-in at the midpoint or end of each session is satisfactory. Most teachers provide feedback at the halfway point, but in long-term groups the individual learners usually want feedback sooner. Group feedback is helpful in several dimensions, prompting the group to reflect on how it is doing and (informally) advising the teacher on what works and what doesn't.

## CONCLUSIONS

Small groups can be an effective modality for learning in all levels of medical education. This modality has a number of advantages because students in groups have a greater sense of ownership and are more active with regard to learning goals, which lead to more meaningful and lasting learning (Westberg and Hilliard 1996). There are disadvantages to small groups, such as higher costs, greater faculty-to-student ratio, greater faculty workload, greater commitment of time for any given learning objective, variable quality of facilitators, variable reliability, and validity of interventions. Evaluation should be intertwined with the objectives—starting up front, rather than after the fact—and linked with documentation such that it facilitates feedback to individuals and the group.

## SMART STRATEGIES

- Find a mentor with interest in group therapy or group learning.
- With your mentor, role-play challenging situations encountered while facilitating group.
- Consider videotaping a session for review.
- Discuss with your mentor your own experiences with good and bad teachers.
- Have fun!

## QUESTIONS TO DISCUSS WITH A MENTOR OR COLLEAGUE

1. How do I know that teaching in a group setting is appropriate for me?
2. What makes a good group facilitator? How is this similar or different from the characteristics of a good lecturer?
3. What opportunities are there locally for me to become more involved in group teaching?
4. Are there organizations that focus on the group modality that I should consider joining?

## REFERENCES

Donner RS, Bickley H: Problem-based learning in American medical education: an overview. Bull Med Libr Assoc 81:294–298, 1993

Westberg J, Hilliard J: Fostering Learning in Small Groups. New York, Springer Publishing Company, 1996

## ADDITIONAL RESOURCES

Crosby JR, Hesketh EA: Small group learning. Medical Teacher 26:16–19, 2004

Dacre JE, Fox RA: How should we be teaching our undergraduates? Annals of Rheumatic Diseases 59:662–667, 2000

Steinert Y: Student perceptions of effective small group teaching. Med Educ 38:286–293, 2004

**Internet resources**

*The following is a comprehensive, well-organized Web site that reviews the key elements of successful small group teaching uses material from David Jaques, an experienced groupwork and teamwork trainer:*

Jaques D: Small Group Teaching [Oxford Brookes University Web site]. Available at: http://www.brookes.ac.uk/services/ocsd/2_learntch/small-group/sgtindex.html. Accessed March 3, 2005.

*This site provides links to other Web resources for small group teaching:*

Keele University: Small Group Teaching. Available at: http://www.keele.ac.uk/depts/aa/landt/links/small_group_teaching.htm. Accessed March 3, 2005.

*This online guide offers practical strategies for improving small group teaching. It contains a nice problem-and-solution section and is well organized and easy to read:*

Soliman I: Teaching Small Groups [Teaching and Learning Centre, University of New England Web site]. Available at: http://www.une.edu.au/tlc/pub/smgroups.pdf. Accessed March 3, 2005.

*This site presents goals, guidelines, and techniques of small group teaching in concise bullet points:*

University of Alabama: Teaching Tips: Small Group Teaching [School of Medicine Web site]. Available at: http://www.uab.edu/uasomume/cdm/small.htm. Accessed March 3, 2005.

*This site presents information and resources for helping educators in all of the health professions enhance their instructional, leadership, management, and research skills, with additional resources that can help with career development:*

University of Colorado Health Sciences Center: Center for Instructional Support. Available at: http://www.uchsc.edu/CIS/index.html. Accessed March 3, 2005.

*The site includes a bibliography on small group teaching:*
http://www.uchsc.edu/CIS/SmGps.html

*and a comprehensive checklist to prepare small group facilitators:*
http://www.uchsc.edu/CIS/SmGpChkList.html

# CHAPTER 17

# Writing Test Questions and Constructing Assessments

Teresita McCarty, M.D.

Assessment is a powerful tool for providing feedback to guide student learning and faculty teaching efforts. It motivates students to learn and encourages them in the practice of lifelong self-assessment. This chapter seeks to guide early career academic psychiatrists in their use of typical assessment methods, types of grading, and approaches to standard setting commonly used in medical education.

Students pay particular attention to the topics faculty members choose to highlight in their questions. Well-chosen questions help students learn.

## TESTING METHODS

All assessment methods have limitations, and no one method can assess all types of knowledge and skills. Any assessment method can be used in either a formative or summative manner. The purpose of a *formative assessment* is to provide immediate feedback during the course so as to guide the student toward any necessary improvements; they tend to be frequent and somewhat informal. The feedback can be given verbally, as a measurement on a scale, as a percentage, or as a written narrative. However the results are conveyed, formative assessment results are not recorded in a student's permanent record. Although a formative quiz or clinical observation may result in a score, the purpose is to give information to the student to guide improvement. *Summative assessments,* on the other hand, tend to be more formal, often occur at the end of a course in order to evaluate knowledge gained by students, and produce a result that is entered into the student's record. This result may be used to make high-stakes decisions such as promotion or graduation. Formative and summative assessments should be congruent in the level of mastery expected.

The three assessment methods that will be described here are as follows:

- Multiple-choice questions, including single best answer and extended matching
- Essay questions, including restricted response or short answer and extended response
- Performance examinations, in which students demonstrate their knowledge and skills

Multiple-choice questions are typically used to measure medical knowledge. Both single best answer and extended-matching multiple-choice questions have been thoroughly researched and are used by the National Board of Medical Examiners on the licensing examinations (Case and Swanson 2002). Essay questions allow students to exhibit clinical reasoning, whereas performance examinations allow students to demonstrate the knowledge and skills necessary for patient interactions. It is important to match the learning objectives with the appropriate assessment method.

## Multiple-Choice Questions

Multiple-choice questions (MCQs) consist of a stem with several associated answer options, only one of which is intended to be the most correct answer. When well written, MCQs have many advantages: they are generally accurate indicators of what the students know; they are efficient in testing a large amount of information over a wide content area in a relatively small amount of time; and they can be scored objectively and rapidly by machine or by hand. However, MCQs also have disadvantages: they are not authentic (patients do not come to us with their problems configured as MCQs); they can inadvertently give students the message that there is an absolute right or wrong answer; they do not tell instructors how students arrived at their answers; and students may choose the correct answer on the basis of a misconception or by guessing.

The strengths of MCQs make them a good place to begin when writing test questions—as long as they are well written and properly used. If you find you cannot write an effective MCQ for a subject, you can always proceed to another assessment method, such as an essay question or performance examination.

## Single Best Answer Questions

Single best answer questions consist of a stem and lead-in followed by a series of three to five answer options, one of which is most correct and three of which are distracters.

**Stem:** When writing the stem, which is the body of the question, remember to focus on important concepts and to aim at the application of knowledge rather than simple recognition or fact memorization. The stem should be as complete as possible, containing enough information that the question could be answered correctly even if the answer options were omitted. The stem should not contain unnecessary information. When the stem consists of a patient vignette, include the patient's age, gender, and the clinical setting along with the presenting symptom and the pertinent history in order to allow the student to answer the lead-in question.

**Lead-in:** The lead-in is the actual question you are asking about the topic or scenario presented in the stem. Write the lead-in question as a complete sentence whenever possible and avoid asking students to answer negatives like "All of the following are characteristics of this disorder *except...*" or "Which of the following are *not...*" Negatively phrased lead-ins are much more difficult for students to read accurately. Recognizing that answers are wrong does not necessarily mean the student knows what is correct, and negatively phrased questions require reading all the options before they can be answered. A well-constructed single best answer question can be answered after reading the stem and lead-in, before looking at the answer options (Figure 17–1, question version 2 only).

**Answer options:** Answer options should be short and should be similar to one another in length and in the type of information they contain. Distracters, the incorrect answer options, should contain common misconceptions and should seem likely to less knowledgeable students. Avoid using absolute terms such as "never" and "always." Just as medicine rarely has absolutely right or wrong answers, you are asking for the *most* correct answer available from the list of options. Avoid nonspecific terms such as "occasionally" and "frequently," because readers interpret these variably. List the options in numeric, alphabetic, or some other logical order and be sure that they are all grammatically parallel with the lead-in to prevent test-savvy students from choosing an option based on grammar clues. Also, avoid "none of the above" and "all of the above" options. These increase the odds of students guessing correctly based on partial recognition of information in the options. The very best students may be penalized when they incorrectly choose "none of the above" because they have come up with a better option than the one you intended to be correct (Case and Swanson 2002).

---

Use the criteria for a well-written single best answer question to evaluate the two questions.

---

Version 1    Which of the following characterizes separation anxiety disorder?

       A. Weight loss, lethargy, loss of usual interests, isolation from others

       B. Excessive hand washing, avoiding cracks in the sidewalk, refusing to eat foods that have touched other foods

       C. Refusing to go to school, fear of leaving the home, anxious when away from parenting figures

       D. Unstable, widely varying moods

       E. Disordered thoughts, affect inconsistent with situation, delusions

Version 2    An 8-year-old boy needs to be coaxed to go to school, and while there he complains of severe headaches or stomach pain. Sometimes his mother has to take him home because of his symptoms. At night, he tries to sleep with his parents. When they insist that he sleep in his own room, he says that there are monsters in his closet. These findings are most consistent with which of the following diagnoses?

       A. Child schizophrenia

       B. Normal concerns of latency-age children

       C. Separation anxiety disorder

       D. Socialized conduct disorder

       E. Symbiotic psychosis

---

**Answer:** Version 1 is poorly written. The question cannot be answered before reading all of the answer options. Version 2 is an NBME example of a well-written question.

---

**FIGURE 17–1.**    Single best answer questions.

*Source.*    (Version 2) Case SM, Swanson DB: *Constructing Written Test Questions for the Basic and Clinical Sciences*, 3rd Edition Revised. Philadelphia, PA, National Board of Medical Examiners, p 49. Reprinted with permission from the National Board of Medical Examiners® (NBME®).

## Extended-Matching Questions

Extended-matching questions consist of a set of questions organized around a list of options. The elements of extended-matching questions consist of a theme, a list of answer options, a lead-in statement, and two or more stems. These questions are very versatile and faculty should be encouraged to write them. The construction tips outlined above for single best answer questions also apply to extended-matching questions. Additional guidelines for constructing extended-matching questions follow.

**Theme:** Identify a set of items that you want to assess. Examples are a set of anatomic locations, a group of medications, or a list of diagnostic classifications.

**Answer options:** Create a homogeneous list of 6–15 answer options related to your theme (e.g., cranial nerves, drugs of potential abuse). The answer options should be brief and listed alphabetically or in some other logical order.

**Lead-in:** Write a lead-in that clearly states the basis for matching the stems or vignettes with an answer option (e.g., "For each patient described, select the most likely drug of abuse"). State whether the answer options may be used more than once (Case and Swanson 2002).

**Stems:** Patient vignettes work very well as stems and should include essential information as described under single best answer questions. Although you may write a stem for each of your answer options, each time a set of extended-matching questions is used in an examination you should have many more answer options than stems. You can use the same set of answer options and lead-in for the next examination but vary the question considerably by choosing a different set of stems. Like single best answer stems, an extended-matching stem should contain enough information that the question could be answered correctly even if the answer options were omitted (Figure 17–2, stems 1 and 2).

## Essay Questions

Essay questions, where the student has to supply the answer rather than choose among possible answers, are especially useful for measuring students' ability to respond without cues, express ideas, and think critically. Multiple-choice questions are too structured to be adequate for these tasks. Essay questions range from short-answer questions where

Use the criteria for a well-written extended-matching question to evaluate the three questions.

**Delirium**

| | | | |
|---|---|---|---|
| A. | Adverse medication reaction | G. | Hyponatremia |
| B. | Delirium tremens | H. | Hypothyroidism |
| C. | Hepatic encephalopathy | I. | Partial complex seizure |
| D. | Hypercalcemia | J. | Sepsis |
| E. | Hyperkalemia | K. | Substance intoxication |
| F. | Hypoglycemia | | |

For each description, select the most likely cause. (Each cause may only be used once.)

1. A 23-year-old previously healthy woman is brought to the emergency room because of acute changes in behavior. She stopped using cocaine 7 days earlier and in the last 24 hours she has had multiple episodes of losing track of conversations, extending her left arm, and dropping things from her left hand. The episodes last seconds to a minute. Afterwards she seems lethargic and answers questions with inappropriate responses that she later does not recall.

2. A 65-year-old man, who for many years drank two six-packs of beer every day, is admitted to the hospital for elective hernia repair. Other than having difficulty sleeping, he is recovering very well until the third hospital day when his blood pressure, pulse, and temperature become elevated. He is also agitated, picks at his bed clothes, pulls out his IVs, and reports visual hallucinations of insects on the walls.

3. Toxic, febrile state resulting from pyogenic microorganisms

**Answer:** Vignette #3 is very limited. Answering correctly requires only simple recall, and the information is not related to a clinical setting in which the recall of such information might be needed.

**FIGURE 17–2.** Extended-matching questions.

the answer is restricted to a word or phrase, to the typical extended-response questions which may require multiple-paragraph answers. For assessment purposes, it is useful to consider a patient progress note as an essay. The disadvantages of extended-response essay questions relate largely to time factors. The time students take to answer essay questions limits the time available for them to be assessed on other topics. The time faculty take to write and validate a key or set of grading standards and then to hand grade each student's answer is also extensive. Therefore, extended-response essay questions should be reserved for assessing critical concepts where faculty want students to demonstrate their thinking and when other methods would be less effective.

To write an essay question, choose important concepts, define a task, and ask students to respond in a manner that demonstrates higher-level reasoning (e.g., evaluation, interpretation, or comparison and contrast). Be clear about your expectations; sometimes providing an example is very helpful for students. While allowing students as much freedom as possible in their answers, be sure to specify pragmatic limits about the number of words and pages, type size, or amount of time permitted.

Short-answer test keys are quite straightforward and consist of a list of the correct answers, whereas extended-response essay question answer keys can be either analytic, assigning points for specific content, or holistic, taking a global approach to quality determination and points earned. Using a clinical progress note as an example, the analytic scoring approach might award two points when the patient's temperature is included among the vital signs. The holistic approach allows the grader to acknowledge that the patient's temperature is sometimes so important that omitting it means the entire note is unsatisfactory. The holistic approach sacrifices some grading reproducibility for greater validity, using an answer key that more closely reflects the complexity of medical reasoning (Schuwirth and van der Vleuten 2003). Whether analytic or holisitic, an essay key outlines the content and style parameters to be assessed and defines the minimum required for each point or quality level. In addition to the key, providing sample essays that represent differing quality levels helps to calibrate or standardize graders. Essay answer keys should be peer reviewed, used on a sample set of student essays, and revised before they are applied after a summative examination.

Whereas short-answer questions are scored by assigning points based on correct responses, essays may be given a single global score or separate scores for criteria like organization and content. It is best to grade essay questions without knowing the identity of the students. Grading the same question for everyone in the group before proceeding to the next question encourages more consistent scoring. One approach is to initially sort the essays into quality groupings (e.g., good, medium, and poor) and then return to each pile to confirm that the essay is correctly placed before assigning the final grade (Gronlund 2003).

## Performance Examinations

Some skills are best measured by having the student physically demonstrate what he or she can do. Watching a student obtain a history, perform a mental status examination, or check reflexes provides a more authentic and therefore more valid skills assessment than asking a student to answer written questions about the same topics. Feedback or coaching provided after a student has been affectively engaged in demonstrating skills has a powerful impact on learning. The Objective Structured Clinical Examination (OSCE) is a type of performance examination that uses standardized patients to improve the fairness and reliability of the outcomes (Hodges et al. 2002). Performance examination disadvantages for the faculty member largely relate to the amount of time needed to write patient cases, train standardized patients, and evaluate the performance as well as the space and money required. Skills-based performance tests are an important complement to knowledge-based tests (Smee 2003).

## STANDARD SETTING

Formal standard setting occurs most frequently in association with summative performance testing and is one of the most important of faculty duties. To set the standard is to decide what examination score indicates that students know enough and perform well enough to progress or graduate. There are many approaches to setting standards, but in general it is a peer group activity that begins with faculty reviewing the curricular learning objectives and the assessment measurement tools (multiple-choice tests, checklists, rubrics, or global scales). Each individual decides on a minimal acceptable score. Because faculty members frequently differ in their expectations, the next step is to discuss the reasoning behind the differing minimal scores. After listening to one another, individuals may choose to revise their initial decision. The final standard is the average of each faculty member's minimal acceptable score (Smee 2003). This process establishes a *criterion-referenced* standard where all students have the opportunity to be successful. It does not necessarily seek to sort students into smaller quality groupings. The use of a criterion-referenced standard may result in all students in a particular group being above (or below) the standard, in contrast to using norm-referenced standards where students in a group are compared with one another. After an examination, the standard should be reviewed to confirm that it was placed correctly; that is, that the students who are below the standard truly did not demonstrate enough knowledge or skill to move to the next step in patient care. In addition to being an important assessment task, standard setting is a wonderful faculty development experience.

Assessment is a powerful tool with which to promote learning in the educational environment (Black and William 1998). Assessments that provide reproducible results (reliable) and accurately measure information or skills that are important to patient care (valid) are measures of learning that are important for students and faculty. Multiple forms of assessment, when chosen to best match a particular knowledge domain or skill set, are a fundamental part of any well-designed curriculum.

## KEY CONCEPTS AND DEFINITIONS

**Assessment:** The act of assigning a value or judgment. In the learning setting, it is the application of a variety of methods that are used to determine if students are achieving intended learning objectives.

**Criterion-referenced standard:** An individual's performance is described in terms of what he or she can or cannot do. The decisions are based on a finite set of criteria and the level of mastery necessary is established by the educators. It assesses whether a particular student achieved the minimal level of mastery, regardless of how the rest of the class scored.

**Formative assessment:** Any learning measure used to provide prompt feedback to the student in order to improve areas of weakness or misconception. Formative assessments are typically informal and administered somewhat frequently.

**Norm-referenced standard:** An individual's score is based on and is described in comparison to the scores of others in a specified group. For example, it may determine that a particular student's score was markedly above the class mean.

**Performance assessment:** A learning measure in which students are required to demonstrate their skills and understanding by performing a task; for example, interviewing a patient, evaluating mental status, or performing a neurological examination.

**Reliability:** The degree to which a student's score within a domain is consistent or reproducible from one assessment to another when the student's ability is unchanged. (Does the assessment arrow hit the same place on the target each time?)

**Summative assessment:** Formal testing used to measure student performance, judge success, and provide documentation for the record. These assessments are typically used to determine competence and assign grades at milestones in the curriculum.

**Validity:** The ability of an assessment tool to truly measure what it is intended to measure. This speaks to the accurate measurement of the meaningful and essential features of the fundamental concepts the students are learning. Asks whether a communications score, for example, adequately predicts how a student communicates with his or her patients? (Does the assessment arrow hit the bull's-eye of the target?)

## SMART STRATEGIES

- Align learning objectives, curriculum learning opportunities, and assessment techniques.
- Administer frequent formative examinations.
- Avoid true or false summative questions.
- Pilot test assessments.
- Peer-review test questions.
- Use a variety of assessment techniques.
- Gather an adequate sampling of student knowledge and performance.
- Establish fair and equitable testing procedures.
- Publicize explicit, specific criteria of what constitutes successful performance.
- Give timely feedback.
- Evaluate assessment methods and revise for quality improvement.

## QUESTIONS TO DISCUSS WITH A MENTOR OR COLLEAGUE

1. How do our residents and students perform on the nationally standardized behavioral science tests?
2. Is our assessment scoring and reporting system consistent with that of the other clerkships, rotations, or training programs?
3. What are the areas in which our assessments could be improved?
4. What variety of assessment methods do we use?
   What is the quality of the measures?
   Do they emphasize what is truly important?

## REFERENCES

Black P, William D: Inside the black box: raising standards through classroom assessment. Phi Delta Kappan 80:139–148, 1998

Case SM, Swanson DB: Constructing Written Test Questions for the Basic and Clinical Sciences, 3rd Edition Revised [National Board of Medical Examiners Web site]. 2002. Available at: http://www.nbme.org/about/itemwriting .asp. Accessed February 18, 2005.

Gronlund NE: Assessment of Student Achievement, 7th Edition. Boston, MA, Pearson, 2003

Hodges B, Hanson M, McNaughton N, et al: Creating, monitoring, and improving a psychiatry OSCE: a guide for faculty. Acad Psychiatry 26:134–161, 2002

Schuwirth LWT, van der Vleuten CPM: Written assessment. Br Med J 326:643–645, 2003

Smee S: Skill based assessment. Br Med J 326:703–706, 2003

## ADDITIONAL RESOURCES

Accreditation Council for Graduate Medical Education and American Board of Medical Specialties: Toolbox of Assessment Methods Version 1.1. [ACGME Web site]. 2000. Available at: http://www.acgme.org/Outcome/assess/Toolbox.pdf. Accessed February 18, 2005.

American Educational Research Association, American Psychological Association, and National Council on Measurement in Education: Standards for Educational and Psychological Testing. Washington, DC, American Educational Research Association, 1999

Chatterji M: Designing and Using Tools for Educational Assessment. Boston, MA, Pearson Education, 2003

Frederiksen N: The real test bias: influences of testing on teaching and learning. Am Psychol 39:193–202, 1984

Jaeger RM: Statistics: A Spectator Sport, 2nd Edition. Newbury Park, CA, Sage Publications, 1993

Mager RF: Preparing Instructional Objectives, 3rd Edition. Atlanta, GA, Center for Effective Performance, 1997

Newble D, Dawson B, Dauphinee D, et al: Guidelines for assessing clinical competence. Teach Learn Med 6:213–220, 1994

Newble DI, Jaeger K: The effects of assessment and examinations on the learning of medical students. Med Educ 17:165–171, 1983

Norman G, Wakefield SJ: Evaluation Methods: A Resource Handbook. Hamilton, ON, McMaster University, 1995

Page G, Bordage G: The medical council of Canada's key features project: a more valid written examination of clinical decision-making skills. Acad Med 70:104–110, 1995

Page G, Bordage G, Allen T: Developing key feature problems and examinations to assess clinical decision-making skills. Acad Med 70:194–201, 1995

Rowntree D: Assessing Students: How Shall We Know Them? New York, Nichols, 1987

Shepard LA: The role of assessment in a learning culture. Educational Researcher 29:4–14, 2000

Zurawski R: Making the most of exams: procedures for item analysis [The National Teaching and Learning Forum Web site]. 1998. Available at: http://cstl.syr.edu/CSTL/NTLF/v7n6/exams.htm. Accessed February 18, 2005.

# CHAPTER 18

# Writing and Reading Letters of Recommendation

Joseph B. Layde, M.D., J.D.

One of the tasks required of every academic in psychiatry or any other field is writing cogent letters of recommendation or support for students, residents, and other faculty members. For an early career academic psychiatrist, learning to write letters that accurately convey the desired degree of enthusiasm for the subject of the letter is something of an art. This chapter describes strategies for writing effective letters that honestly convey information about their subjects as well as your level of enthusiasm for them without running afoul of laws pertaining to confidential information.

## MAKING YOURSELF AVAILABLE

It is a good idea for young academic psychiatrists who teach to make it known that they are available to write letters of recommendation for medical students and residents whom they know well and whose accomplishments they can fairly describe in a letter. Attending psychiatrists in medical student clerkships have an excellent opportunity to observe students' clinical skills firsthand. Whether a student is applying for a residency position in psychiatry or in another field, a letter of recommendation from an attending physician who has worked closely with him or her can be very useful to residency admission committees in evaluating applicants for their programs. Similarly, attending psychiatrists who supervise residents in inpatient or outpatient rotations can provide useful insights into the clinical acumen and work habits of residents looking for a fellowship position or a job.

However, it is also important for you to be willing to tell students or residents that you cannot write an effective letter if you feel that you do not know enough about their clinical work. Similarly, it is only fair for you to give students and residents a general idea of the tone of the letter that you would write; you should be honest about telling poor students and residents that, while you would be willing to write a letter of recommendation for them, you could not wholeheartedly recommend them. Professional integrity mandates that you not write untruthful letters of uncritical support for mediocre candidates. What's more, over time, institutions and colleagues get a feel for the credibility of your letters of recommendation and support. Your letters will be most persuasive if you develop a reputation for not overselling or underselling the qualifications of their subjects, but rather for accurately portraying them.

In the United States, the federal Family Educational Rights and Privacy Act, also known as the Buckley amendment, prevents an educational institution from disclosing personally identifiable information from a student's education record without the student's written consent. Therefore, it is important to receive written consent if you plan to include information such as a student's grades in a letter of recommendation. However, opinions of a student's work or his or her ability to perform in a particular role are not, strictly speaking, part of the student's educational record; the Buckley amendment does not require written consent for their disclosure. Most medical schools have a "Consent to Release Academic Information" form available for medical students to sign that explicitly gives the school and its faculty members permission to include educational records in letters of recommendation. In addition, many students will sign a waiver of their right to inspect letters of recommendation. It is generally thought that residencies give more credence to letters of recommendation that are accompanied by a statement that the named student has waived his or her right to review the letter, presumably allowing the candid expression of the author's opinions about the student's character and performance.

## BEING TRUTHFUL

One of the most difficult tasks for new academic psychiatrists to master in writing letters of recommendation is that of truthfully describing any negative qualities of its subject. For instance, you may be asked to write a letter for a medical student whom you sincerely like, but who you think lacks the requisite self-knowledge to succeed in a psychiatry residency. How should you handle the situation? First, you should counsel the student about career choices. If you think psychiatry is a poor career choice for the student, you should explain your reasons for feeling that way, making clear that you like the student as a person. If the student decides to apply for a psychiatry residency anyway and asks you for a letter of recommendation, you should be honest about what you plan to say in such a letter. You can tell the student that you would accurately portray him or her as affable and academically gifted, for instance, but that you would include a mention of an apparent lack of introspection and how you believe that would affect his or her career as a psychiatrist. Given that information, the student would most likely go on to ask someone else for the letter of reference. However, if the student desires the letter nonetheless, stick by your guns and include the information you said you would include.

Another difficult situation comes up when you are asked to write letters of support for faculty members who are coming up for promotion or tenure; the task may include evaluating the candidate against a set of criteria established by his or her institution. In this situation you may not have the opportunity to tell the candidate of your misgivings about whether he or she meets the criteria because such letters are typically requested by the Rank and Tenure Committee of an institution, which may specifically request that you not discuss the letter with the candidate. Honestly listing the pros and cons of a candidate's achievements as they relate to the criteria of the candidates' institutions requires objectivity, but it is essential for making the promotion system work.

## BEING SPECIFIC

Residency programs evaluating medical students, medical practices considering hiring graduating psychiatry residents, award committees determining to whom they will grant the award, and institutions considering promoting faculty members all want specific information in letters of recommendation or support.

A generic letter of recommendation that blandly states that "Jane Smith was a capable and friendly medical student and a pleasure to work with" is unlikely to sway a residency admission committee very much. The addition of details helps make the subject of the letter come alive and gives the reader a much better picture of how the applicant might function in a new position.

A letter of recommendation should start out with an explanation of how you have worked with the candidate. For instance, "I am delighted to write a highly enthusiastic letter of recommendation for Jane Smith, who is a fourth-year medical student in my institution. I have known Ms. Smith very well for four years, having served as a small group leader for her first-year problem-based learning group in the Foundations of Human Behavior course. I also served as the clerkship director and team leader at the VA Medical Center Psychiatric Inpatient Service where Ms. Smith was one of four students rotating through the third-year psychiatry clerkship in the fall of 2003." Such an introduction establishes the fact that you have worked closely with the candidate and have been in a position to know her strengths and weaknesses. It also establishes that your letter gives a longitudinal picture of the candidate, rather than just a snapshot.

Tailor your letter to the specific purpose at hand. For instance, when writing a letter of recommendation for a medical student for a psychiatry residency program, explain in what ways the student's performance in medical school demonstrated the requisite intellectual skills, sense of professional responsibility, and communication skills needed in a good psychiatric resident. When writing a letter of recommendation for a graduating psychiatry resident seeking his or her first clinical position after residency, emphasize characteristics of the applicant likely to be important to the hiring practice, such as ability to get along well with patients and staff members, completeness of medical record documentation, and timeliness and dependability throughout his or her residency. Readers of a letter will appreciate learning how the applicant is likely to perform in the specific role for which he or she is being considered.

Whenever possible, and always taking into account the requirements of the Buckley amendment, describe how the subject of your letter stands out. An effective letter of recommendation for medical student Jane Smith might contain the following paragraph: "I have been the site director of the psychiatry clerkship at the VA Medical Center for the past six years and have had nearly 200 students work with me during their third-year clerkships in psychiatry. Ms. Smith is certainly one of the five most outstanding students I have worked with during that time. Her communication skills with patients on the ward equaled that of an excellent third-year resident in psychiatry, and she gave a superb brief oral presentation of her review of the literature on tardive dyskinesia on patients on atypical antipsychotics to our team. She scored at the 98th percentile nationally on the National Board of Medical Examiners Subject Examination in psychiatry at the end of her clerkship." The specifics listed about Ms. Smith's performance on her rotation clearly get across to the reader the reasons why the letter writer thinks she would be an excellent psychiatry resident. The data behind the letter support the enthusiasm the writer is conveying. Useful data to put in a letter include the following:

- A ranking of the candidate among trainees you have worked with
- The number of trainees you have worked with
- How long you have been working with trainees
- Externally produced information like standardized test results

## WRITING WITH STYLE

Letters of recommendation and support should not be wordy. A three-page letter of recommendation that lacks specific information about the candidate is of much less assistance to the reader than a one and a half page letter that specifically describes how the candidate meets the criteria for becoming a fine resident, assuming the responsibilities of an early career clinician after residency, receiving a teaching award, or being promoted to associate professor at his or her academic institution. Letters of recommendation will not be any good to the subject or to the reader if they are full of jargon or turgid prose. Use simple, declarative sentences, with quotations when appropriate. For example, a letter of support for a faculty member you are nominating for a national teaching award can be livened up by including verbatim quotations from medical students' or residents' evaluations of the faculty member's teaching: "Dr. Adams made psychiatry so compelling to me during my third-year clerkship with him that I am now looking seriously at psychiatry as a career. He is an excellent role model." The enthusiasm of the third-year student for the teaching of Dr. Adams will stand out when the awards committee deliberates on the choice of winner.

Make sure that you have access to all of the useful information about the subject of your letter. Often, a curriculum vitae does not highlight the most relevant attributes of a candidate. When you are writing a letter of recommendation for a medical student, it is important to have available to you the student's grades, the dean's letter, and any descriptive comments made by clerkship directors. (Again, remember to only include that information if you have a signed release permitting the disclosure of academic information.) If you are writing a letter of support for a faculty member for a national award or for promotion, it is important that you have access to institutional data on the faculty member's evaluations by medical students or residents, recent research projects, institutional awards, and publications. Wherever possible, get copies of recent scholarly articles written by medical students, residents, and faculty; this allows you to include a well-informed judgment of the candidate's scholarly achievements in your letter. Table 18–1 presents a checklist for writing a letter of recommendation or support.

## ALLOWING FOR FURTHER COMMUNICATION

It is a good idea in letters of recommendation and support to include a final paragraph such as the following: "Thank you very much for your attention to my letter of support for John Andrews, M.D., Ph.D., for his consideration for the National Teaching Award of the American Association of Psychopharmacology. If this selection committee would like further information, I can be contacted by telephone at (414) 555–2387." Including such a statement allows the reader of the letter to contact you to clarify specific points in the letter if necessary. Some admission committees and employers like to confirm the contents of written letters of recommendation with a telephone interview. Even if you are not contacted by the reader of your letter, your inclusion of an invitation to call shows that you stand behind it.

## READING LETTERS OF RECOMMENDATION AND SUPPORT

You may often be the recipient of letters of recommendation for applicants for residency, candidates for new faculty positions, and nominees for awards. Be as discriminating in reading those letters as you are in writing them. Look for evidence in a letter that the writer personally knows the attributes of the person he or she is writing about—look to see how long and in what capacity the writer has worked with the subject of the letter. You are likely to give much more weight to a letter that specifically describes an applicant's performance in a relevant area of expertise—for example, her performance as a fourth-year medical student taking an elective on a VA psychiatric consultation service—than in one that blandly characterizes her as "a fine student."

Notice if a letter you are reading omits some obviously relevant detail. For instance, does a letter about a residency candidate in psychiatry go on at length about the degree of scientific knowledge that the candidate possesses, but make no mention of the candidate's skill in dealing with people? The author may be eloquent in what he or she does not say about a candidate, and by careful reading one can discern important information from glaring omissions.

---

**TABLE 18–1.**    Checklist for writing a letter of recommendation or support

---

- Gather evaluations of medical students, residents, or fellow faculty members for whom you are writing the letter.
- If appropriate, inform the subject of the letter of the general tone that your letter will carry.
- Obtain written permission to release educational records, if applicable.
- Organize information so you can write clearly, specifically, and succinctly.
- Quote evaluations verbatim.
- Close the letter with an invitation to the reader to contact you for more information.

---

If the author put forth the invitation, and if you would like more information about the subject of a letter, call the writer and ask for clarification. Over time, you will come to rely on dependability of some of your colleagues' letters. Put a great deal of stock into letters written by those you know and trust and from whom you have received a variety of letters, showing a variable degree of enthusiasm for candidates of varying degrees of qualifications.

## SMART STRATEGIES

- Make yourself available to medical students, residents, and other faculty members as someone who is willing to write clear letters of recommendation and support.
- Get written permission to disclose the educational records of students for whom you write letters of recommendation.
- Use verbatim quotes from evaluations to make letters of recommendation and support more specific and lively.
- Close letters with an offer to give more information by telephone.
- Keep the following in mind when writing letters of recommendation or support: truthfulness, specificity, relevance, clarity, and succinctness.

## QUESTIONS TO DISCUSS WITH A MENTOR OR COLLEAGUE

1.  What are the most important characteristics of a young physician to include in letters of recommendation or support for positions in residency programs, early career jobs, nominations for national awards, and applications for promotion or tenure?

2. How does a letter writer best provide an unvarnished portrait of the subject of the letter, including his or her strengths and weaknesses?
3. When writing letters of support for academic physicians seeking promotion or tenure at an institution other than your own, how do you evaluate a candidate's credentials for promotion or tenure at the other institution?

## ADDITIONAL RESOURCES

Aamodt M: Predicting performance with letters of recommendation. Public Personnel Management 22:81–90, 1993

Beller JM: Accountability, honesty, and recommendations. Strategies 11:33–36, 1997

Brown LL: Fourteen ways to write a better letter of recommendation. Professional School Counseling 3:141–146, 1999

Hartzell GN, Nelson K: Writing for dollars: composing recommendation letters. School Counselor 40:312–315, 1993

Jones DW: College letters of recommendation. School Counselor 38:153–155, 1990

Kaplan R: Faculty references: how to offer an opinion on a student's ability to work. Journal of Career Planning and Employment 5:12–13, 1994

Palmer SE: What to say in a letter of recommendation. Chronicle of Higher Education 27:21–22, 1983

# PART V

# Developing Your Academic Skills...

# CHAPTER 19

# Searching the Literature to Find the Information You Need

Cynthia M.A. Geppert, M.D., Ph.D.

Each day a flood of new information comes to psychiatrists' mailboxes and computers: journals, conference announcements, book catalogs, e-mail alerts, article digests, and news updates. An early career academic psychiatrist can feel as if he or she is drowning in data and often will wonder where to find the time amid clinical, teaching, and family responsibilities to stay current with the literature. Gone are the days of lectures, textbooks, exams, and syllabi that offered so much more clarity and direction on important material to be mastered. This chapter is intended to help in navigating the ocean of information that currently exists (Geppert 1998); it will explain basic search strategies for the major databases used in psychiatry, demonstrate how to locate significant government and institutional reports on mental health, and provide practical advice about how to keep up to date with important discoveries in psychiatry.

## DATABASES

Like everything else in informatics, the number, complexity, and types of databases have grown exponentially. Fortunately, there are just two main databases with which the early career academic psychiatrist needs to be familiar: PubMed and PsycINFO. The characteristics of these are summarized in Table 19–1.

**TABLE 19–1.**   Databases

| Database | Characteristics |
|----------|-----------------|
| PubMed | • Web-based retrieval system developed by the National Library of Medicine<br>• Database of life sciences bibliographic information<br>• 15 million citations dating back to the 1950s<br>• Links to full-text articles and third-party sites |
| PsycINFO | • An abstract (not full-text) database of psychological literature from the 1800s to the present<br>• Available through libraries and a variety of proprietary information services<br>• 2 million citations and summaries of journals, books, chapters and dissertations<br>• Covers psychology and related disciplines |

## SEARCHING THE DATABASES

Most clinicians have had the discouraging experience of trying to search for an article on a specific topic in MEDLINE, the National Library of Medicine database for life sciences and biomedical bibliographic information, and being overwhelmed with 5,000 citations! Try to view this as a blessing in disguise. PubMed, MEDLINE's free and public interface, employs "MeSH" terms, the controlled vocabulary used to index articles for consistent retrieval of information. PubMed uses the "explode" approach: it casts a wide net and uses the subcategories of the hierarchical MeSH system to retrieve articles that can be useful when you want to know what is generally available on a broad topic (Doig and Simpson 2003; Ebbert et al. 2003; National Library of Medicine 2004). The MeSH approach is crucial to successful searching because the novice searcher does not need to master the taxonomy of the National Library of Medicine. PubMed will match the search terms to similar concepts that may use different terms. For instance, if you put in the words *manic depression*, you will obtain related citations on bipolar disorder, depression, manic disorder, and so on.

More often, a psychiatrist seeks the answer to a specific clinical question or information to accomplish a scholarly task. Efficient search strategies exist that were originally geared to PubMed but can be adapted to almost any database. Three useful PubMed strategies to hone in on specific topics are 1) limits, 2) related articles, and 3) Boolean logic.

PubMed has a "Limits" dropdown feature that enables you to narrow

**TABLE 19–2.** Boolean logic

| Term | Logic | Example |
|------|-------|---------|
| AND | Retrieves a set of articles each of which contains each search term, without regard for order. | Posttraumatic stress disorder AND acute stress disorder |
| OR | Retrieves a set of articles each of which contains at least one of the search terms. Provides a set of articles on similar subjects. | Posttraumatic stress disorder OR acute stress disorder |
| NOT | Excludes retrieval of the designated term; may eliminate relevant articles. | Posttraumatic stress disorder NOT acute stress disorder |

the search by using a variety of filters. Some of the most helpful are language, age, publication or entry date, and human or animal. For a search on new addictions pharmacotherapy information to be used in a lecture, for example, select the limits of "English" and "human," and set the date of publication to the last 3 years. Two other limit categories can further refine retrieval. "Publication Types" locates particular kinds of articles, including clinical trials, editorials, letters, meta-analyses, reviews, practice guidelines, and randomized, controlled trials. "Reviews" and "practice guidelines" would provide the kind of overview information required for the lecture assignment. Under "Subsets" is the category of *bioethics* that could focus a search for citations pertinent to writing a paper on confidentiality protections in psychotherapy.

A second strategy can be used once the results of your search have come up: the "Related articles" link (found next to each citation) locates references related to the original article by comparing words in the title and abstract, as well as MeSH headings, to other citations. This is useful when a search retrieves few articles on a topic (Doig and Simpson 2003; Ebbert et al. 2003; National Library of Medicine 2004).

A third strategy is to employ Boolean logic (see Table 19–2), a system that uses the operators "AND," "OR," and "NOT" to symbolize relationships between terms and thus guide searches. Note that these operators must be capitalized to work (National Library of Medicine 2004).

## HOW TO SEARCH PUBMED STEP BY STEP

**Step 1:** Go to the PubMed Web site (Figure 19–1). Many university library home pages have a link to PubMed, or you can insert the URL listed below.

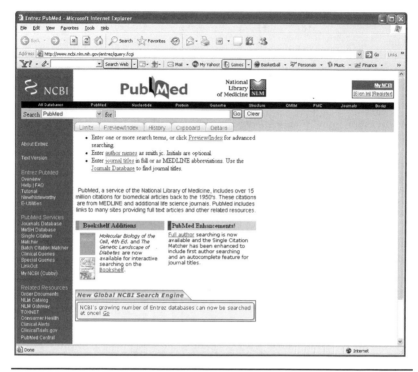

**FIGURE 19–1.**    Main search page of PubMed.

*Source.*    From: http://www.ncbi.nlm.nih.gov/entrez/query.fcgi.

It is a free site and open to the public: http://www.ncbi.nlm.nih.gov/entrez/query.fcgi.

**Step 2:** Say you have a patient with posttraumatic stress disorder who has terrible nightmares and you want to learn about evidence-based treatments for nightmares. In the "Search PubMed For" box, type *posttraumatic stress disorder*. You receive 8,773 citations and feel completely overwhelmed. Don't panic. You need to narrow and focus your search just as you would do when trying to solve any clinical question. Apply the Boolean logic you just learned.

**Step 3:** Return to the "Search PubMed For" box and type *posttraumatic stress disorder AND nightmares*. You receive 219 hits. This seems much more manageable, but it is still a lot to go through when you have clinic in an hour. Now is a good time to use the limiting feature explained above to further narrow your search and reduce the number of citations.

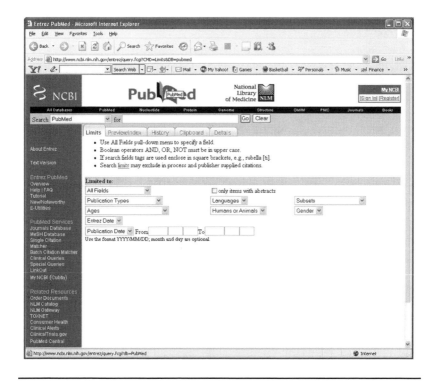

**FIGURE 19–2.**   Limits feature in PubMed.
*Source.*   From: http://www.ncbi.nlm.nih.gov/entrez/query.fcgi, after selecting the "Limits" feature button at the top of the pane.

**Step 4:** Using the pull-down menus, select "Languages" and choose
"English." In the "Humans or Animals" menu, choose "human." Rerun
your search and you drop the number of citations to 200—still more
than you can review before the patient arrives. Therefore, let's assume
that you are only interested in literature from the last 5 years when evidence-based medicine was more widely utilized, and you further decide that you only want to see randomized, controlled trials.

**Step 5:** Return to the "Limits" feature screen (Figure 19–2). In the box
that reads "Publication Date," enter the parameters of interest to the
years 2000–2005. This reduces your citations to 67. You may then hone
in on what you want to know even more closely by choosing the "Publication Types" pull-down menu and selecting "randomized controlled
trials." You now have six citations on your topic of interest.

Now you can look more in depth at each article. Usually there is an abstract, and often, more recently, publications will offer a free full-text version of the article that can be downloaded.

## FINDING GOVERNMENT AND INSTITUTE REPORTS

The political and social aspects of psychiatric practice are increasingly important and visible. To stay abreast of research and policy developments, early career psychiatrists must know how to quickly locate salient government and scholarly reports and other types of documents. Two widely quoted sources are reports of the Institute of Medicine (http://www.iom.edu/reports.asp) and of the Surgeon General (http://www.surgeongeneral.gov/library/reports.htm). Often clinicians will spend hours searching for core statistics on mental illness epidemiology and mental heath services. Excellent U.S. government resources for this kind of information are the National Institute of Mental Health (http://www.nimh.nih.gov), the National Institute on Drug Abuse (http://www.nida.nih.gov), the National Institute on Alcohol and Alcoholism (http://www.niaaa.nih.gov), and the U.S. Department of Health and Human Services' Substance Abuse and Mental Health Services Administration (http://www.samhsa.gov/index.aspx).

## STAYING CURRENT

No one can possibly read every interesting psychiatric journal article or keep abreast of the rapid pace of discovery in the neurosciences. Yet continuing education is an ethical mandate of our profession. Several tools are available that review and analyze high-quality literature and present it in accessible form. *The New England Journal of Medicine* publishes *Journal Watch Psychiatry*, which offers physician-authored summaries and commentary on clinically important articles and the latest research breakthroughs compiled from major psychiatric and general medicine journals. Another such tool is PsychLinx, part of the MDLinx network. (MDLinx is a company that employs physician editors to sort articles and research from more than 2,000 peer-reviewed journals daily into 34 medical specialty sites online.) PsychLinx is a proprietary technology aggregate that produces daily e-mail newsletters with highly focused content dealing with topics such as substance abuse, psychopharmacology, and mood disorders. Hundreds of peer-reviewed articles in top categories are scanned and categorized with complete bibliographic information. These tools should not be used as a substitute for reading original articles and primary sources but rather as a guide to pertinent and timely publications.

## SMART STRATEGIES

- Become familiar with PubMed and one other database and develop proficiency so that you can locate articles on a specific topic in 10 to 15 minutes.
- Formulate a plan to regularly review practice guidelines from the American Psychiatric Association and other major organizations.
- Use your continuing medical education requirements to maintain general psychiatry knowledge outside your specific area of practice.
- Transform academic assignments such as lectures and presentations into opportunities to acquire modest expertise in a new area of psychiatry.
- Construct a systematic strategy of staying current by using a combination of printed and electronic resources, and integrate this plan into your daily or weekly schedule.
- When important reports are issued, invest the time to locate them, thereby learning about new information resources.

## QUESTIONS TO DISCUSS WITH A MENTOR OR COLLEAGUE

1. Can you help me perform a targeted literature search using PubMed?
2. Do you have an efficient strategy that you can share with me for staying current with important literature?

## REFERENCES

Doig GS, Simpson F: Efficient literature searching: a core skill for the practice of evidence-based medicine. Intensive Care Med 29:2119–2127, 2003

Ebbert JO, Dupras DM, Erwin PJ: Searching the medical literature using PubMed: a tutorial. Mayo Clin Proc 78:87–91, 2003

Geppert CM: Rescuing the doctor: swimming lessons for physician-educators. Otolaryngol Head Neck Surg 118:423–428, 1998

National Library of Medicine: PubMed Tutorial [PubMed Web site]. July 2004. Available at: http://www.nlm.nih.gov/bsd/pubmed_tutorial/m1001.html. Accessed March 3, 2005.

# Evaluating Clinical Research Studies

Teddy D. Warner, Ph.D.

Donald M. Hilty, M.D.

Clinicians and scholars alike are rightly taught that they must keep up with the latest developments in practice and research. However, the volume of potentially relevant materials to read and evaluate—or even just scan—can be daunting. One must consider general medical journals (e.g., *Journal of the American Medical Association*), specialty journals (e.g., *American Journal of Psychiatry*), and subspecialty journals (e.g., *Academic Psychiatry*). However, keep in mind that not all articles should be given equal scrutiny. First, you must decide what you need to get from the article and how much effort to apply to make your reading more efficient. The depth to which you read the article depends on five main purposes for which psychiatrists use literature: 1) in search of general knowledge; 2) in search of new ideas to apply to clinical care, education, or research; 3) to gather general background material in order to design a new study or grant proposal; 4) to gather the most directly relevant data as background to write a manuscript that reports their own original research; and 5) to gather systematic data about the state of the literature in some area in order to write a review article.

It is impossible to be a first-rate researcher, educator, or academician without devoting the necessary time, skill, and motivation to read, understand, and critically appraise primary literature (also see Chapters 19, 21, 22, and 24). However, doing so is arduous, not only because of the volume of literature but also because of the increasingly sophisticated research now published using more complex data-collection methods and data-analysis and interpretation approaches. Journals today include a wide range of types of articles: reports of empirical studies such as clinical trials; articles that review the empirical literature in an area; conceptual or theoretical pieces; opinion or editorial writings; letters to the editors, which may include important critiques of prior published empirical studies; reviews of professional books; and a variety of other writings. Our purpose here is to give you a general approach to reading and critically appraising journal articles that report empirical studies (i.e., the primary literature), and then an approach for more broadly assessing the literature pertaining to some phenomenon as a whole.

## BACKGROUND

Think about your goals in going through stacks of publications or electronic materials. For example, if you need an authoritative report on standard treatments in order to teach your trainees fundamental ideas, a review article or book chapter might be good. If you want cutting-edge data for clinical care, you will not mind the limitations inherent in a group of case reports. If you are writing up the results of your latest study, you will need to understand (and cite) the current state of the most directly relevant published knowledge. If you are a leader in your field and writing a review article, you will need to read and carefully evaluate all the relevant published articles—an abstract will not suffice.

It is sometimes helpful, rather than simply reading the primary literature, to focus on secondary sources of information found in review journals, society newsletters, textbooks, or commercially recorded media. This approach is much more efficient, requires less mastery of complex methods and data, and relies on experts. A disadvantage to this approach lies in the filtering process, which introduces an additional and potentially major subjective element into the evaluation. For practice issues, the bias of others tends to be corrected with enough time, but researchers generally must know the current state of knowledge and accepted methods, even though these also will evolve over time. Many studies are open to varying interpretation, and reliance solely on others puts one at a distinct disadvantage at times, particularly where scholarship is concerned. Summaries of studies done by others do not convey the nuances of methodological or analytic approaches or their strengths and weaknesses the way reading the primary literature does.

## ANATOMY OF AN EMPIRICAL ARTICLE

It is essential that you understand what you should expect from each part of an empirical article. You are most likely familiar with the six standard components of empirical articles used in most sciences today (abstract, introduction, methods, results, discussion, references; see Chapter 22 in this volume), and you should approach reading any article with these components in mind to organize or structure your reading. The most coherent processing of articles requires that you first gain a general understanding of the study from a careful reading of the *abstract*. If that convinces you that the article is of importance to your practice or research, then proceed with an analytic reading of the main sections of the article body. While reading these sections, it is important to be rationally critical, but fair, asking yourself the questions listed in Table 20–1.

Skilled readers report that they selectively read various sections of the article in different orders. However, a simple sequential reading of all sections is always appropriate if you are confident that the article is of considerable relevance for your practice or research. Certainly, you can never fully and fairly evaluate an article and the study it reports without a full and careful reading of the entire article. Keep in mind that relying on colleagues, associates, or assistants to digest articles for you has some of the same disadvantages of relying on experts in secondary sources, except that your associates and assistants are not nearly as likely to be as informed and critical as experts are. Thus, there is no avoiding appraising primary literature directly if you desire a real appreciation and full understanding of the published literature.

Once your careful reading of an abstract tells you that you should critically evaluate the entire article, begin with an assessment of the *introduction* section. The introduction should give you a clear review of directly relevant, previously published literature. In a report of an empirical study, this section should not be expected to review the entire relevant literature but only what is most pertinent to the present study. It is the purpose of review articles, not empirical reports, to describe and discuss large extant literatures. Of course, if you are not an expert in the area being studied, you will not likely know whether or not the article adequately discusses and cites the most important and germane literature. However, a careful analysis of the literature cited and briefly discussed in the introduction should give you a feel for whether or not the introduction succeeds in placing the current study in the appropriate context. From the discussion of relevant prior studies, the article should directly move toward how the present study will add to that literature,

**TABLE 20-1.**   Criteria for evaluating clinical research studies

1. What are the quality and the reputation of the journal in which the article is published?
2. Is the title clear and informative?

**Abstract**

3. Are the purposes, hypotheses, study population, sample, study design, primary outcome measures, main results, and main conclusions and implications of the study clear in the abstract?

**Introduction**

4. What is the type of article (e.g., full report of a clinical trial, a brief report, a pilot study)?
5. What is the main objective of the study? Will meeting the objective enhance understanding in the field or subfield?
6. Does the introduction adequately discuss and cite the literature that is centrally important to the study? Does the article discuss superfluous literature not germane to the purpose of the study?
7. What are the primary hypotheses, if any, and are they clearly stated in a testable form? Are there secondary hypotheses? Are the hypotheses reasonably justified and significant to the field?

**Methods**

8. What population is sampled for the study? What is the theoretical population of interest (i.e., about whom do the researchers ideally wish to generalize conclusions)? How is the sample drawn (e.g., randomly, purposively, self-selected)?
9. What type of study is it—descriptive, correlational, quasi-experimental, or experimental?[a] What is the full study design using information about the independent variable (see item 10 below) and the type of research design?[b]
10. What are the main independent or predictor variables (if it is not purely a descriptive study)? Are the independent variables important or peripheral to the phenomenon under study? Are independent or predictor variables manipulated by the researchers, or are they only measured as attributes of participants? How many levels or categories of each independent or predictor variable are there? Is the independent variable a *between-subjects* variable[c] or a *within-subjects* variable[d]?
11. What is the level of measurement of the predictor, independent, and dependent variables (nominal/categorical, ordinal, interval/continuous, or ratio/continuous) and are the analyses suitable for that level of measurement?

**TABLE 20–1.**    Criteria for evaluating clinical research studies *(continued)*

12. What is the main dependent or outcome variable or variables? What is the level of measurement of the dependent or outcome variable(s) (*nominal/ categorical, ordinal, interval/continuous, or ratio/continuous*) and is the analysis suitable for that level of measurement? Are there primary outcomes on which the study focuses and also secondary outcomes that are less central to the effects of the independent or predictor variable? Were the most conceptually important outcomes measured?

13. Is there sufficient evidence for reliability and validity of main outcome variables and predictor variables (none, provided by the present study, provided by past literature based on citations)?

14. Are outcomes measured by accepted state-of-the-art measures (this is preferable), or are they assessed by new measures developed for the current study? Are the outcome measures conceptually the most appropriate ones?

15. What level of control (i.e., *randomization, stratification, equivalent groups, statistical control*) is exerted in the study over extraneous variables (i.e., variables other than the independent and dependent variables)? Do any important uncontrolled extraneous variables produce possible confounds with the independent or predictor variables that might provide alternative explanations for study results?

16. Does the methods section adequately describe key features of the study such that the study could be replicated by others and that you can fairly assess the likely validity of results?

**Results**

17. At the outset of the study, are groups that are compared in the study equivalent or different on important characteristics that might be related to the outcomes or influenced by the independent variable or predictors (i.e., can preexisting characteristics or conditions explain or confound the study results)?

18. What is the dropout rate of study participants, and does this vary by study group? How does this compare to other studies of its type using similar approaches? Did sufficient numbers of study participants complete the final study outcomes to provide adequate statistical power?

19. Is there sufficient statistical power to detect the smallest effect sizes that are clinically meaningful?

20. Are appropriate statistical procedures applied to the data? Were important assumptions for these procedures met? Would alternative or additional statistical procedures add to the ability to understand results?

21. Does the results section clearly and succinctly describe all important results in the study based on the objectives and hypotheses? Were clear and informative tables of data included?

**TABLE 20–1.**    Criteria for evaluating clinical research studies *(continued)*

**Discussion**

22. Does the discussion section clearly and succinctly summarize the major results from the study, the important implications of the study results, the important limitations of the study, and needed directions for future research?

23. Are the study results appropriately interpreted (i.e., was interpretation justified by the nature of the measures, how they were obtained, who they were obtained from, and how they were analyzed)? Were conclusions appropriate, overstated, or misleading?

24. What is the overall assessment of internal validity of the results of the study (i.e., how confident are you that the results obtained are valid reflections of the study hypotheses or objectives)?

25. What is the overall assessment of external validity of the results of the study (i.e., to what degree can the results be generalized to the theoretical population of interest and to real-world situations)?

26. Do the study results contribute to the existing knowledge base (i.e., current relevant empirical literature) incrementally? If not, is the study so novel that it provides unique information? Do the study results replicate or contradict important previous findings? Do study results have practical or theoretical relevance?

27. Based on an overall evaluation of the article, does the research seem valid? Do you believe the results? If not, what is your rationale for not believing the results?

28. What research should follow from this work, and did the authors discuss it?

**References**

29. Are all citations included in the body of the article cited in the reference list? Are they cited in standard fashion such that they could easily be located in the literature?

---

[a]Types of study design: *descriptive* (e.g., case studies and simple survey results), *relational* or *correlational* or *associative* (e.g., complex self-report and surveys), *case-control* or *quasi-experimental* (i.e., pre-existing groups that are equivalent or non-equivalent), *experimental* (i.e., randomized groups), or a combination of these.

[b]Example of a research design: *Treatment Group* ( control vs. drug A vs. cognitive-behavior therapy) [between subjects], × *Time* (baseline vs. endpoint vs. 3-month follow-up) [within subjects] × *Disorder Severity* [continuously measured].

[c]A between-subjects variable is represented by different groups of individuals.

[d]A within-subjects variable is repeatedly measured at different points in time (most commonly), or measures from different sources that are correlated (e.g., from husbands and wives as pairs).

conceptually, theoretically, and practically. At this point you should be able to understand the reasons why the study was conducted.

After the purpose of the study is explained, the research hypotheses usually follow. Sometimes there are no hypotheses in strictly descriptive studies, such as case reports or observational studies. However, even in exploratory or pilot studies, the investigators surely have some ideas regarding how the data are likely to turn out and should be willing to state so at least in general terms.

The third component of empirical articles is the *methods* section, which describes how the study was actually conducted. Although this section is avoided by many readers, experts will often tell you to read this section first (following the abstract) because the methods include the substance of the article, especially the part that must be carefully analyzed and evaluated to determine the likely validity of study results. The new information obtained from a study is only as good as the methods are sound. Therefore, the core of your appraisal must be the methods section. Were state-of-the-art procedures and techniques used? If not, were the alternative procedures adequately justified? Perhaps it is the case that the work is so novel that it is not clear what the state-of-the-art procedures might be, or maybe current procedures in an area are known to be deficient and the current article improves on them. Do such innovative approaches provide valid data—data that move the field forward—or is the innovation simply superficial? It is the design, the methods, and the analyses of data in an article that determine the overall worthiness of the work, regardless of what might be a wonderful literature review or a clever discussion. It is on the methods and results sections that you should focus your appraisal as a scientific critic— a different emphasis from that of the prepublication reviewer or the author, both of whom must focus on all parts of an article.

The methods section may or may not provide a general description of the *design* of the study (including the main independent or predictor variables); this description is sometimes presented at the end of the introduction or omitted entirely because of the simple nature of the study. The methods section should describe the sample of people who participated in the study, the population from which they were drawn, and how they were drawn. The methods should also describe the major outcome variables (dependent or criterion variables) and show how the data were collected. That is, measures should be briefly described in such a way that the reader might obtain, use, or reconstruct them for another study. Likewise, a description of procedures used in the study must be included in sufficient detail, as well as a description of any intervention process, so that others may attempt to replicate the study. (However, do not expect excessive detail that is unrealistic or burdensome to describe.) In medical journals, the last part of the methods section is often a brief description of statistical procedures applied to the major outcome variables. Often, casual readers skip reading the methods, especially the procedures—but to fairly evaluate a study, an appreciation of all aspects of the methods is essential. It is only by evaluating how a study was actually conducted that the appraiser can determine whether or not results are likely to be valid. Otherwise, your trust is entirely in the authors, the reviewers, and the editors.

The *results* section presents the data obtained through execution of the study methods. Analyses and description of the data are presented in prose, tables, and figures; footnotes to tables and figures often include information essential for complete understanding. Different journals have varying approaches as to whether information in tables and figures is also described in the text. Various journals also have different styles regarding the amount of detail that is used to describe statistical procedures and results, but more is generally better if you want to evaluate the work. If insufficient detail is provided in the results section, it is probably due to the particular journal style and should not negatively affect your evaluation of the study. If you need more detail (because you are attempting to conduct related replicating or extending work or writing a review, for example), you can e-mail or write to the corresponding author of the study. Results also often include some modest interpretation of the data, but substantial interpretation is left for the discussion section.

*Discussion* sections often begin with an overview of study results manner that is somewhat redundant with the results section but uses less technical language and goes into much less detail. In this section, results of the study should be placed in perspective and compared with the existing knowledge in previous publications, and a reasonable interpretation of the direct results should be offered. Consistency and differences with what is known should be discussed. Some speculation within limits is permissible, but judgment must be exercised to prevent going too far a field from what the data might reasonably support. Alternative explanations to study findings posited in the introduction or elsewhere should be mentioned. Major flaws or limitations of the study are also listed in this section, as are particular strengths of the work, especially if its methods, approaches, or samples go beyond those that have been used before. Finally, it is common to end with suggestions for future research that would extend or improve the present study and other published work.

The list of *references* completes the article. An appraisal of the work must include careful examination of the reference list, something that most readers avoid. First, consider whether key citations from the literature are missing and whether the authors have adequately described the work of others in the introduction and by giving credit in the reference list. Ideally, this list should provide readers with the general background that is needed to become familiar with the phenomenon and begin a study on their own. However, as indicated above, if the area is well developed and a large body of literature exists, the reference list must necessarily be selective and include only the seminal works in the area and others that are most directly related to the current study. An author can certainly cite too few past works but also can cite too many, unless a literature review article is the object of the appraisal. Such a review article should, of course, discuss and cite every article pertinent to the defined scope of the review and explain why certain articles or types of articles were excluded.

## ASSESSING THE LITERATURE

After your efforts to assess individual articles as described above and in Table 20–1, you may be confronted with the task of assessing multiple published articles all bearing more or less on the same issue. You may need to do this to have a general sense of the state of knowledge, or for clinical practice considerations, or for more focused scholarly purposes, such as designing your own studies or writing reviews of the literature. It is unlikely that all relevant articles in an area lead clearly to the same conclusion (although sometimes they do). How do you assess the whole picture? The literature probably includes some conflicting results and certainly includes studies that have varying characteristics and methods, even if they have the same general objective (such as examining whether cognitive-behavioral therapy [CBT] is effective for treating depression and whether it is more or less effective than certain drugs).

If you are fortunate, recent articles that review the relevant literature have been published by experts in the field, and you can simply accept their conclusions. However, sometimes multiple reviews exist that have reached somewhat different conclusions or have focused on different aspects of the phenomenon. Of course, you may wish to consult textbooks and other scholarly books (especially edited volumes) to gain an overview of the phenomenon of interest. However, realize that textbooks have limitations different from those of the primary literature—they are 2–4 years behind the literature, they tend to make conservative conclusions that do not reflect even emerging literature at the time they are published, and they certainly make global pronouncements that may be far less useful than more specific primary articles in particular contexts. If you are skeptical of existing textbooks, or if reviews or such sources are not available, then you will need to assimilate the literature yourself.

One of two methods is usually used to conduct literature reviews to assess what the published literature indicates about some phenomenon. The first and oldest approach, still commonly used, is mainly descriptive (Fink 1998). The reviewer counts features of studies (e.g., number of studies that achieve high rigor vs. those that do not; number of studies published by year or decade). Using informed judgment, the reviewer interprets trends related to study findings and conclusions as a set (e.g., 65% of all studies found CBT effective for treating posttraumatic stress disorder; 87% of studies in the past decade found CBT effective). This descriptive approach is more or less what researchers do (with widely varying quality) when composing the introduction or background sections to their articles. Of course, descriptive reviews of trends are fraught with great potential for bias, although such reviews have made and continue to make very important contributions to the literature by systematizing sometimes quite extensive and diverse literatures.

In contrast, meta-analytic reviews (or meta-analyses) are evaluations of the literature based on quantifiable characteristics of each individual study using inferential statistics to reach conclusions about those studies as a group. The raw data (observations) for a meta-analysis are the quantified results of each study (i.e., the study is the unit of analysis, rather than study participants as in primary literature). Specific characteristics of articles are coded as variables (e.g., nature of the sample, such as male vs. female or severely ill vs. mildly ill), sometimes with judgments being made about specific elements of the study (e.g., strength of controls on a scale of 1–5). Most importantly, the summary statistic that represents the size and direction of the effect (e.g., Cohen's $d=0.62$ and Pearson correlation $r=0.45$ are common effect-size measures) of the independent or predictor variable in published studies is assessed as the prime dependent variable in a meta-analysis. With inferential statistical procedures, the effects across all reviewed studies are assessed for magnitude and reliability (i.e., whether there is evidence for a reproducible effect of the treatment, for example, across 23 studies for which mean $r=0.37$, $P<0.01$). The coded characteristics of the studies are used as independent variables in the meta-analysis to determine if various features of studies influence the reliability or magnitude of the effect in the studies. The technical aspects of conducting such reviews are far beyond our scope here (Hunter and Schmidt 2004).

For assessment of the literature, however, neither practitioners nor researchers will likely perform a meta-analysis to assess the literature unless they plan to publish such a review. Instead, descriptive review procedures are likely to be used in everyday evaluations of the literature. At the first level of analysis, you will simply want to assess the pattern of direct results or conclusions of the various articles (e.g., 73% of studies found regular use of vitamin E is correlated with number of cardiovascular events). In such reviews, you will then need to assess the methodological features of each article, much as we recommended above. You are likely to select several key features (e.g., dose level) as most important based on your understanding of the literature, realizing that it would be very difficult to systematically and individually assess even most of the 29 items listed in Table 20–1 for an entire study. Of course, in writing the review, you will weigh studies with greater methodological rigor as more likely to be valid. You will likely find that even though study objectives were similar, outcome measures differed across the studies, and even that the specific nature of the independent variables differed (e.g., different dose levels, treatment durations, or treatment qualities). Overall, what is the pattern apparent in the literature? How can you apply the pattern of findings to your practice or to your own research? Your informal or formal literature review should focus on notable strengths of the literature as whole as well as significant weaknesses, without focusing on trivial flaws of published studies.

## FINAL EVALUATION OF A PUBLISHED WORK

The final decision about the value of an article or set of articles rests with the consumer, which is you, the reader, as practitioner or competing scientist. Often, however, readers as appraisers are too passive and are intimidated by the power of the printed word, especially if it is found in prestigious journals. Who are we to criticize the journal editor, the peer reviewers, and the authors themselves? Presumably, all are experts. But keep in mind that the burden of proof is on the authors and publishers to convince us of the validity and usefulness of the work. Each reader must make an independent assessment, recognizing, of course, that his or her analysis too may be flawed.

If you are a critic, be aware that it is very easy to reject a published article (or a manuscript being reviewed) as unsound and it is essentially impossible to find flawless work. All studies have weaknesses, and you must be suspicious if a study presents results without common confounding events, particularly in studies that were difficult and expensive to execute. There are many more ways a study or any complex endeavor can go wrong than can go right. This is not to say that scientists should not have high standards and expectations, but that they must always keep those in perspective.

## SMART STRATEGIES

As you are evaluating clinical research studies, ask yourself the following questions:

- Having appraised (rather than merely read) the article, do I generally believe the study results and conclusions? If not, what are my reasons for disbelief?
- What novel and nontrivial contributions to the literature do the study results make?
- Do I understand how the study results fit with other published work and knowledge?
- How might I remedy any study weaknesses (e.g., in biostatistics, research design, or sampling) if I were to undertake the study myself?
- What plausible alternative interpretations are there for the study results?

## QUESTIONS TO DISCUSS WITH A MENTOR OR COLLEAGUE

1. Should I participate in a journal club to assess literature with peers (or lead one for trainees)?
2. How can I expand my access to literature through Internet searches and sources?
3. Which journals and listservs are essential reading in our field or subfield?
4. What implications do recent published empirical studies have for my practice?
5. What are some important questions that could be answered by research that I might be currently prepared to conduct?

## REFERENCES

Fink A: Conducting Research Literature Reviews: From Paper to the Internet. Thousand Oaks, CA, Sage Publications, 1998
Hunter JE, Schmidt FL: Methods of Meta-Analysis: Correcting Error and Bias in Research Findings. Thousand Oaks, CA, Sage Publications, 2004

## ADDITIONAL RESOURCES

Ascione FJ: Principles of Scientific Literature Evaluation: Critiquing Clinical Drug Trials. Washington, DC, American Pharmaceutical Association, 2001

Gelbach SH: Interpreting the Medical Literature. New York, McGraw-Hill, 2002

Roberts LW, Geppert CM, Brody JL: A framework for considering the ethical aspects of psychiatric research protocols. Compr Psychiatry 42:351–363, 2001

# CHAPTER 21

# Publishing a Manuscript

Alan Louie, M.D.

John H. Coverdale, M.D., M.Ed., FRANZCP

Kristin Edenharder, B.A.

Laura Weiss Roberts, M.D., M.A.

The ability to communicate effectively is central to science and to academic success. Your publication record is the metric of your contribution to the field, which is relative to national (or, in some cases, international) standards of scholarship. Other parts of your resume are important, but promotion committees will want to know how many articles you have published in peer-reviewed journals, preferably as the first author. One may contribute to academic literature with various types of manuscripts, including original research articles, commentaries, review articles, book chapters, book reviews, and annotated bibliographies. This chapter will focus on original research manuscripts, for the practical reason that empirical articles are most likely to provide academic recompense.

## DATA-CENTERED MANUSCRIPTS

Original research manuscripts are data centered (see Chapter 20 in this volume and Table 21–1 for a detailed discussion of the anatomy of an empirical article). This has three implications: First, the manuscript will be only as good as the data on which it is based. Many writers are more motivated to write about their ideas than about their data. These priorities should be reversed for original research writing. Think first about what data you will publish and then think about the concepts that they may support. If the data do not meet your standards, then you should continue working to gather more. The second implication is that you do not need to publish all of your data. You may feel that every piece of data is like your child; however, not all of it is going to be publishable. Pick the best-quality data. The third implication is that the data dictate the focus and conclusions of the manuscript. Reassess your research questions and the scope of your study in light of the information ultimately obtained, and don't draw conclusions that your data do not support. For the conclusions you propose, note any caveats resulting from the study's limitations.

## GETTING PUBLISHED

Publishing a manuscript is like selling a product. It must be assessed, properly packaged, and strategically placed in the right market. With a manuscript, the first step is to assess its contribution to the field. How significant are your findings to the field at this time, and who will be interested? What is the quality of your data and the rigor of the underlying methods? How much competition is there from other manuscripts on the same topic? The answers to these questions will determine how you package your manuscript and will direct you in choosing an appropriate target journal for submission.

### The Right Format

How you package your manuscript relates to the type of article you will submit. Journals allow different types of research manuscripts—for example, letters to the editors, brief reports, original articles, and special articles. In that order, they range from approximately 500 to 4,500 words. Check the journal's Web site for author instructions and their exact manuscript specifications. Because space is always at a premium with journals, the longest format is reserved for manuscripts with the most significant findings and the most rigorous science. Shorter formats may be used for pieces that present less significant findings but still merit publication because they explore new avenues of research or describe some innovation. As an author, you will need to assess at which level to submit your manuscript. If you submit a special or original article, the reviewers will expect more and be more critical. The editors may respond with a rejection, but it is also likely that they will suggest that the article be scaled down to a shorter format. Thus, all may not be lost, but resubmission in a shorter format will require re-review by the journal and can greatly extend the publication timeline.

| **TABLE 21–1.** | Key elements of original research papers |
| --- | --- |

**Structured abstract**

Approach this section last.

Serves as a complete summary of manuscript, usually read first by readers.

Follow specifications of target journal for appropriate length and format.

**Introduction and references**

Indicate the significance of your research question.

Note how your study will answer important questions.

Note why your study is needed at this time.

Provide a balanced review of the literature, including studies for and against your position.

**Method**

Establish validity of the study.

Describe treatment and comparison conditions, the data collection process, and analytic procedures.

Provide sufficient detail to allow replication.

Be sure statistics are appropriate, clear, and reasonably explained.

**Results**

Present the results in both text and tables.

Present data in a concise manner, don't repeat data in both the text and tables, and leave out extraneous details.

Be sure the data in the text and tables are not contradictory and that the numbers add up.

Present data in a clear manner; your most dramatic findings should be graphed.

Present explanations and speculation about the data in the discussion, not in the results.

**Discussion**

Note the limitations of your study.

Only draw conclusions that are clearly supported by your data.

Indicate the contribution of your study and the future research for which it has set the stage.

## The Right Journal

Targeting the right journal increases your chance of acceptance. If you are totally off base in your submission, the editor will return your manuscript before even sending it out for peer review, with an indication that it is not appropriate for the journal. Assuming the editor does take your manuscript under review, your topic may or may not be one in which the journal has particular interest. Even if your manuscript is solid, the editor's decision about publication is discretionary, merely because there is limited space for which many good manuscripts compete. Your topic may fall within the general purview of the journal, but the editors may be focusing on other themes and topics at any given time. A quick way to assess the current trends of a journal is to read the abstracts and articles published in the last several issues. Also look for announcements in the journal calling for papers on specific topics. You may also wish to contact the editors and ask them if your manuscript would be appropriate and encouraged by the journal. In addition, it is important to assess whether or not the manuscript is generally competitive with other submissions to the journal. Sometimes this relates to the rigor of the data. For instance, some journals are mainly interested in randomized, controlled trials or will only take survey studies with high response rates.

Finally, as with most things in academics, there exists an unofficial hierarchy of journals. Some suggest that authors aim high by submitting to the most prestigious journals and going elsewhere if rejected. While this strategy has its merits, it is important to be realistic. Indiscriminant submission of manuscripts that will mostly likely be rejected causes delay in the ultimate publication date and is abusive of the editorial review process.

## The Right Audience and Impact

Deciding if your manuscript and a journal are a good match is up to not only the journal's editors but you as well. Your objective is to communicate your findings to a particular group and to as many people in the group as possible. Therefore, you want to determine the audience and the impact score of journals you are considering. Impact scores are available for several journals and are usually based on how often the journal is cited in the scientific literature. You also want to get your message out in a timely manner. The most prestigious journals, because they receive so many high-quality manuscripts, often have the greatest delay between the submission date and publication date, which may be as long as a year. This may not be acceptable to your timetable as you seek dissemination of your work or academic promotion. You should initially consider a wide list of possible journals. Formulate a list of potential journals by looking at 1) the journals in your references, 2) the American Psychiatric Association's synopsis of journals, and 3) computer searches for journals with articles on your topic.

Having chosen the type of article and the journal, you are ready to submit your manuscript. In this crucial step, be sure to format the manuscript according to the instructions provided to authors by the journal. Editors don't appreciate nonconformity in this regard, and if the manuscript is in the format of another journal, it is a tipoff that your paper was rejected by that other journal. Common errors include not structuring the abstract, not indicating the word count, and not citing references in the correct style. Editors abhor wasting space in the journal, so shorten and be concise wherever possible. Lastly, proofread carefully and have a mentor critique your manuscript. Remember that when you have been so close to your work for so long it is hard to see, or accept, its deficiencies.

## DEALING WITH THE EDITORIAL REVIEW PROCESS

The most important advice to remember is not to take the review process personally. Reviewers are colleagues who volunteer their time to improve the quality of the psychiatric literature. Reviewers generally feel they are expected to provide constructive criticism, even for the best manuscripts. Look at the reviews as free advice from experts in the field. Reviewing manuscripts is a subjective process, and reviewers frequently do not agree. If you are confused by what the reviewers say, look to your mentor to help you interpret the reviews.

The reviews will be accompanied by a cover letter from the journal's editors. The editors will have weighed the input from all the reviewers and will have come to a decision about your manuscript, which is expressed in the letter. The decision is usually acceptance, rejection, or something in between. Most often it will be in the last category, which will require some revision of your manuscript, as suggested by the reviews. The wording of the letter should give you some idea of the chance your manuscript has of being published after revision. For instance, they may say that they look forward to publishing your manuscript if you make revisions, or they may only agree to re-review it with revisions. In the latter case, you have no assurance that it will be accepted after revision, and you should decide whether to resubmit the manuscript to the journal or to send it to another journal.

Authors will usually decide to revise a manuscript and resubmit it rather than start all over with reviews at another journal. Remember that it is a small world, and the second journal might coincidentally use some of the same reviewers you had the first time. When you are ready to resubmit your manuscript, include a cover letter that outlines each of the reviewers' suggestions, indicating that you have carefully considered them all, and address how you have changed the manuscript with respect to each suggestion or why you have chosen not to make the change. It is important that this letter be detailed, yet easy to read.

The editors will review your revised manuscript and may send it back to the original reviewers or to new reviewers. Thus, a second round of comments on your manuscript, now revised, is collected by the editors. This may again result in acceptance, rejection, or something in between. In the latter case, the editors may ask for further revisions, usually indicating that the first revisions did not go far enough. This iterative process could go on indefinitely, but the editors will usually reach an acceptance or rejection decision after the first or second revision. Navigating the editorial review process requires persistence, determination, and a willingness to accept criticism and work with the journal through the revision process.

Ultimately, the best way to understand the editorial process is to see the other side and to be a reviewer. For a preview of this perspective, see the chapter on manuscript reviewing in this volume (Chapter 22).

## ETHICS IN WRITING

Your manuscript should reflect adherence to ethical standards set for research and publishing. For instance, one should address the issue of informed consent when research subjects are involved. Approval of your research by an institutional review board should be noted.

The reporting of one's data must conform to the ethics of scientific researchers. Data should be graphed in a manner that does not distort or hide important aspects of the data. The authors are responsible for applying appropriate statistics to the data and seeking the help of a statistical consultant if necessary. Lastly, one should not selectively suppress data that are inconsistent with one's thesis.

Determination of authorship is another area presenting ethical issues. Authorship denotes credit, and credit should be given only if it is due. Omit honorary authors who do not substantively contribute to the manuscript but are included for political reasons or as quid pro quo. Authorship denotes responsibility for the data and assertions put forth by the manuscript. Authors should not be included who are not willing to assume this responsibility. Also, the final list of authors and the order of authorship on the byline can result in conflict between colleagues. Authorship should be discussed up front as the research is formulated and then revisited as the research is executed. The expected contribution from each author should be made clear, with the order of authorship determined by the degree of contribution. Don't wait until you are about to submit the manuscript.

## GETTING HELP

One of the best places to begin in search of publication help is with a mentor. He or she will provide advice based on experience as well as moral support. Junior faculty members should be wary of joining any department in which they cannot identify potential mentors (see Chapter 26 in this volume). If necessary, one may be able to work with a mentor outside one's institution, usually someone met at a national meeting.

Look for writing workshops given at your institution or at national meetings. Ask your mentors and friends to read your manuscripts and to be frank with their comments. Some authors do best with a writing partner; if this is your case, seek someone with complementary writing strengths.

Scholarly writing requires time and energy and may seem slow and laborious. Factors that can inhibit writing include a lack of confidence or time, an attitude that the writing must be perfect, and a concern that the research is not important enough. Confidence in writing follows, in part, from an attitude that you are the right person to be writing on the topic at a particular time and from an appreciation of how the research contributes to knowledge, even if only in a small way. Further, it is often helpful to start with the methods section, because this simply describes what was done in sequence by the researcher. The method is relatively easy to write and, along with the statement of goals or purpose, sets up the writing of the results.

Several variables might be considered relevant to writing efficiently. These include choosing a personal workspace that is relatively free of distractions where you have been able to work effectively previously. When time is limited, a relatively effortless method for composing an early draft is to write as if you were spontaneously presenting to a colleague. Also consider abiding by a fixed-ratio schedule for writing by taking a break (as one form of reward) after a prescribed number of words or paragraphs or a specific section of the manuscript has been completed. In this way, regular productivity can be assured. Writing with a colleague is a smart strategy that can reduce barriers to writing, add to the fun of the process, and contribute to the quality of the outcome.

## YOUR PUBLICATION RECORD

Remember that promotion committees are going to look at your overall publication record (see Chapter 4). They will look for quantity and quality; that is, how many first-authored publications you have in peer-reviewed journals. Some authors focus too much on one of these factors to the exclusion of the other. The quantity-focused authors have the gift of gab on paper. They need to monitor the substance of their manuscripts and consider consolidating their work into a manuscript for a prestigious journal. The quality-focused authors are great perfectionists, never publishing until the data and writing are impeccable. They need to consider writing manuscripts in parallel, some for prestigious journals and some for less prominent journals.

We all hope to publish one of those seminal articles that will stand out like a beacon, but you cannot count on that. More realistically, you should hope to have a couple of articles that make it into the most prestigious journals. Usually you will also have a variety of publications in good, but less prestigious, journals. While these may not be thoroughbreds, they may be the workhorses of your publication record. Sometimes they are the building blocks for a larger work, or they serve to confirm your previous studies or to reframe your general thesis. Some of your publications will serve to provide balance and breadth to your record, showing that you have published on diverse topics in various journals.

In sum, don't forget the bigger picture. Periodically check the health of your publication record in terms of quantity, quality, balance, diversity, and direction. Formulate an informal 5-year plan for increasing and developing your publication record. For most of us, writing and publishing are hard work with no up-front guarantees, but keep trying, and keep writing! You are likely to find your efforts rewarded by the critical reformulation of your ideas that writing often entails and the benefits of sharing your work with colleagues.

## KEY CONCEPTS

1. Scientific writing is a specific type of writing that is data-centered; the quality of the manuscript is limited by the quality of the data.
2. Each journal has different expectations concerning acceptable data and manuscripts; you need to become aware of these expectations before making a submission.
3. Editorial review of your manuscript is a process, often a protracted and interactive one. Actively managing and negotiating the review process is a learned, professional skill.

4. Remember that your data and ideas have impact only if people read about them. You have to push yourself to publish.
5. If your publication record is a forest, each article is a tree. Don't get lost in the trees. Attend to the overall growth, direction, diversity, and balance of your cumulative publication record.

## SMART STRATEGIES

- Explore your writing inhibitions.
- Realize that the best manuscripts are rewritten multiple times before they are ever submitted.
- Seek out a writing partner or mentor.
- Don't take negative reviews personally; always respond professionally.
- Learn how and what the journals and your audience want you to write, not what you want.
- Keep submitting your work and keep writing.

## QUESTIONS TO DISCUSS WITH A MENTOR OR COLLEAGUE

1. How can I clarify my academic goals and the role writing plays in my professional development?
2. What are my strengths and weaknesses in writing, from your perspective?
3. How can I get helpful feedback on my writing?
4. What is the best way to handle criticism of one's writing?
5. What is the best way to improve one's writing skill?

## ADDITIONAL RESOURCES

Borus J: Writing for publication, in Handbook of Psychiatric Education and Faculty Development. Edited by Kay J, Silberman EK, Pessar L. Washington, DC, American Psychiatric Association, 1999, pp 57–94

Callaham ML, Knopp RK, Gallagher EJ: Effect of written feedback by editors on quality of reviews: two randomized trials. JAMA 287:2781–2783, 2002

Coverdale J, Louie A, Roberts LW: Getting started in educational research. Acad Psychiatry 29:14–18, 2005

Jefferson T, Alderson P, Wager E, et al: Effects of editorial peer review: a systematic review. JAMA 287:2784–2786, 2002

Jefferson T, Wager E, Davidoff F: Measuring the quality of editorial peer review. JAMA 287:2786–2790, 2002

Joint Task Force of Academic Medicine and the GEA-RIME Committee: Review criteria for research manuscripts. Acad Med 76:899–978, 2001

Kazdin AE: Publication and communication of research findings, in Research Design in Clinical Psychology, 3rd Edition. Edited by Kazdin AE. Boston, MA, Allyn and Bacon, 1998, pp 451–466

Mitchell JE, Crosby RD, Wonderlich SA, et al: Elements of Clinical Research in Psychiatry. Washington, DC, American Psychiatric Press, 2000

Roberts LW, Coverdale J, Edenharder K, et al: How to review a manuscript: a "down to earth" approach. Acad Psychiatry 28:81–87, 2004

# CHAPTER 22

# Serving as a
# Manuscript Reviewer

Thomas Heinrich, M.D.

Peer review is the process by which editors rely on experts to advise them on the academic value and scientific merit of manuscripts submitted to their journals for publication. Therefore, peer review plays an important role in determining what is published and what may subsequently become part of scientific literature. Publications in peer-reviewed journals are one of the many factors that contribute to academic promotion and stature (see Chapter 11 in this volume). Expert peer reviewers help to ensure that authors meet the ethical and scientific standards of excellence necessary for publication in today's scientific journals. Peer review has provided standards for publication in academic literature for over a century (Burnham 1990).

Establishing expertise in a field of study is an important factor in founding an academic reputation and seeking professional advancement in academia. Early career physicians can help others to accomplish this goal by serving as respected, expert peer reviewers. Unfortunately, thoughtful reviewing of scientific manuscripts and literature reviews is an academic skill often ignored in postgraduate training. As a result, early career faculty may be at a loss when it comes to reviewing the scientific work of peers. Ideally this skill is learned with the help of a skilled and patient mentor. This senior colleague may invite you, with the journal editor's permission, to help review a submitted manuscript and may then evaluate your completed review. Some journals assign a junior reviewer to each manuscript, allowing a more senior reviewer to tutor the junior colleague. Junior faculty may also learn the trade by reading the peer reviewers' comments on their own manuscripts—an all-too-often painful lesson. The goal of this chapter is to provide a practical framework from which to start the process of learning how to serve as an expert reviewer.

## THE PUBLICATION PROCESS

When an article is submitted for publication, to the novice author it may seem at times to have entered a type of black hole, not to be seen again until months later. However, as is shown in Figure 22–1, the editorial and publication processes are relatively consistent across journals and involve many systematic steps.

Articles submitted for publication to a journal are first screened by the editor for general relevance to the journal, importance of the topic, and general quality. Manuscripts deemed potentially appropriate for publication are then sent to the author's peers for a review. These peer reviewers, or referees, are considered experts in the manuscript topic area, and their names are generally retained in a reviewer database for the journal. The number of external reviews solicited by the journal varies. On average, a manuscript is reviewed by two to four peers, although the number may depend on the journal or type of manuscript. Reviewers, ideally, provide the editor with documentation of both the strengths and weaknesses of the paper. The editor then uses these reviews to inform his or her decision on whether the manuscript is appropriate for publication. The editor, not the reviewer, makes the final publication decision about acceptance or rejection.

## WHAT MAKES A GOOD REVIEWER

There is little empirical evidence as to what makes a good reviewer. The basic quality of idealism is fundamental to a good referee (Goldbeck-Wood 1998). A strong sense of academic and social responsibility, coupled with a desire to teach in a collegial manner, is also very important. Editors look for reviewers who are knowledgeable, can write clearly, and are constructive in their criticisms (Steinecke and Shea 2001). Scientific studies have found that there is little association between the demographic characteristics of reviewers and the quality of reviews produced (Black et al. 1998). However, one study may be reassuring to early career faculty, in that it found that younger reviewers actually produced better-quality reviews. In this study, there was also a negative, but statistically nonsignificant, relationship between academic rank and review quality (Evans et al. 1993).

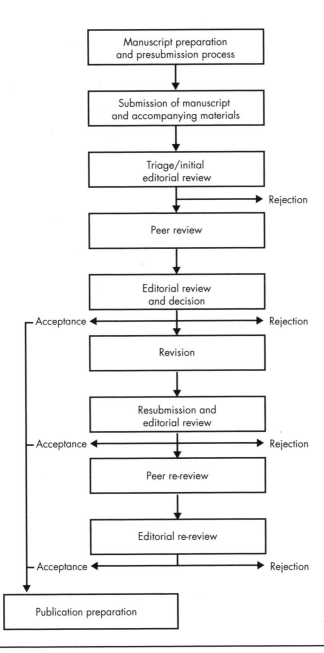

**FIGURE 22–1.** The editorial and publication process.

*Source.* Reprinted with permission from Roberts LW: "How to Review a Manuscript: A 'Down-to-Earth' Approach." *Academic Psychiatry* 28:81–87, 2004. Copyright 2004 *Academic Psychiatry*.

## HOW TO REVIEW A MANUSCRIPT

### Request to Review

The editors select reviewers by matching the manuscript topic with a reviewer's area of expertise. Reviewers are usually selected from a database (compiled by the editorial board) of experts in particular fields of study. Potential reviewers may be queried through several mechanisms, including e-mail or regular mail, depending on the journal. Journals also differ in whether or not the identity of the manuscript's author is made known to the reviewer. The possible reviewer is given the option to either accept or decline the invitation to review. Potential reasons to refuse the offer to review include a conflict of interest, inability to commit the appropriate amount of time to the review, and a lack of expertise in the manuscript's topic (Roberts et al. 2004). If a review is declined, one may be asked by the editor to identify another potential reviewer. Journals differ in the amount of time allowed reviewers to complete their task. It is important that reviewers recognize these time constraints and use due diligence to meet these deadlines. If unable to finish the review in the allotted time, one should let the editors know as early as possible so another reviewer can be selected. The author's manuscript is given to the reviewer in confidence. The manuscript's contents should not be discussed with others until publication.

### Preparation

The time one spends preparing to review a manuscript can be invaluable. How one goes about preparing varies considerably from individual to individual and from manuscript to manuscript. The ability to commit an appropriate amount of time to the review is an important consideration. One must often read a manuscript multiple times before feeling comfortable with the privilege of reviewing, and potentially criticizing, the author's hard work. The time required to conduct a good review varies considerably depending on the type of study, and the length and quality of the report. One study showed that quality of reviews improved with time spent up to 3 hours, but not beyond (Black et al. 1998). Also in preparation, individuals may wish to obtain relevant recent publications in the manuscript's area of focus providing them with an awareness of the current literature (Hoppin 2002). This review of the pertinent literature is often quite helpful, as it frames the paper relative to current publications. A quick read of the abstract and report ideally orients the reviewer on the general direction and purpose of the paper and helps focus the following critical read.

## The Critical Read

Your assessment of a manuscript will depend on the nature and goals of the paper. For example, refereeing literature reviews, case reports, and scientific manuscripts will require slightly different skills sets and points of view. Literature reviews need to focus on the importance, relevance, usefulness, accuracy, and completeness of the literature summary. Clarity, fairness, and a complete representation of the questions and issues important in the area of work that is being summarized are crucial (Roberts 2002). Reviews of case reports focus on the relevance of the case to the journal's readership along with an appropriately detailed summary of the case and sufficient literature review. Rationale for the author's conclusions coupled with potential alternate explanations are further important considerations. Reviews of research studies focus on the problem statement, literature references and documentation, relevance, research design, statistical analysis, results, discussion, and conclusion (Bordage and Caelleigh 2001).

The referee should focus on the quality of the science, regardless of the type of manuscript. In research reports this may include the application of scientific principles and methods. The introduction of the report should build the case for the importance of the manuscript and relevance to the reader. The research question must be phrased clearly and concisely (McGaghie et al. 2001) and, again, the research must be relevant to journal's readers. There is significant competition for publication in academic journals, therefore determining the importance and relevance of topic is imperative for the journal's editorial board. The research design must be appropriate for the research question posed. The design should be described in significant detail to be replicated (McGaghie et al. 2001). The statistical tests performed should be appropriate to answer the research question. If the reviewer feels unable to comment on the statistical tests utilized in the report, it is appropriate to report this and subsequently request a specific statistical review by someone more experienced in the statistical tests applied. The results need to be presented rationally and completely with a clear structure. Agreement among tables, figures, and text is imperative to avoid confusion (Regehr 2001). The conclusions of the study should be clearly stated and must be based on the reported results and potential alternative explanations and study limitations should be discussed (Crandall and McGaghie

2001). There should be no conflict of interest apparent in the study. Note of the institutional review board's approval should be made for studies involving human subjects (Pangaro and McGaghie 2001). The references to scientific literature should be up to date, complete, and appropriate to the topic discussed. Whenever possible, references should refer to the original or primary research papers (Crandall et al. 2001).

For both empirical reports and literature reviews, the peer reviewer must also comment on the presentation style. The report must have a logically organized structure, and the text should be well written without the inappropriate use of jargon or abbreviations. Units of measure need to be consistent, just as tables and figures should appear appropriate and accurate. Literature citations need to be complete and pertinent, allowing a reader to quickly obtain relevant referenced articles.

## Recommendations and Etiquette

There is an expectation of professional courtesy and a clear etiquette in performing reviews. The reviewers should take a collegial and collaborative view towards the process, avoiding harsh or derogatory language and focusing instead on positive comments and, when appropriate, constructive criticism (Roberts et al. 2004). When writing critiques, the reviewer must function as a colleague or coach by offering suggestions for improvement truly intended to help the author. Even if the reviewer's ultimate recommendation is that the scholarship is premature and the paper should be deferred or declined, the aim should be to assist the author in preparing better, more sophisticated work. The role of the reviewer, then, involves both generativity and evaluation. The reviewer is not the ultimate decision-maker. The responsibility for accepting, rejecting, or recommending revision of a manuscript resides within the role of the editor who must decide, based on feedback and guidance from multiple reviewers who may have seen different strengths or weaknesses of a particular manuscript. The resulting collaborative and, hopefully, collegial experience of the review process may help the early career reviewer find comfort in the sometimes daunting task of passing judgment on a fellow academician's hard work.

## Communication of Findings to the Journal

Documenting your thoughts as a reviewer often takes three forms: 1) a journal-specific review form, 2) comments to the author, and 3) confidential comments to the editor. Different journals utilize different review forms to help the reviewer quantify their findings. Various scales may be provided by the specific journal to structure a reviewer's assessment of the science and its presentation in the article. Most journals will have a section on their forms that will provide space for substantial narrative comments for both the author and the editor.

In terms of the narrative response, most written reviews are modest in length (1,000–1,500 words) and the reviewers' identities are masked. A reviewer's comments to the journal often begin with a brief summary of the manuscript describing the topic, scientific approach, major findings, and conclusions. A clear statement by the reviewer regarding the paper's significance is a key element in the review. This is followed by a description of weaknesses and strengths in the paper in its present form; specific examples here are more helpful than broad generalizations. Weaknesses should then be followed by concrete suggestions for potential means of improvement or correction. The potential value and strengths of the paper should be identified. This is followed by specific questions raised during the course of the review regarding the content and presentation of the paper. Suggestions for improvement may be made in a collegial manner. It is here that reviewers often serve as educators to their peers.

Comments to the editor should be relatively brief and should offer direct and specific guidance of special value to the editor. For example, this is a place where the reviewer may give emphasis to the value of the work—or, on the other hand, of the effort and challenges that may be required in improving the work. It may simply be a quick summary of the paper's important points as the reviewer sees them. Finally, it may be a place where the reviewer indicates the limits of his or her expertise and the need to have an additional review performed (e.g., statistical or research design). Editors read these pithy comments to gauge the reviewer's bottom line on a particular paper and to determine whether they have obtained the feedback and guidance needed to do a fair appraisal of the scholarship.

## CONCLUSIONS

Peer review is an important part of the institutions of science and medicine, and it is a valuable skill for the academic psychiatrist to acquire early in his or her career. The quality of the scientific articles reported in medical journals depends on the quality of the science submitted, the performance of the reviewers, and the editorial decisions of the journal's editorial board. Therefore, the training of competent peers to review the work submitted is in everyone's interest: author, editor, clinician, scientist, and patient. Reviewing a peer's hard work is an honor and a privilege. Reviewers have the ability to teach their peers, as well as learn from them.

## SMART STRATEGIES

- Prepare appropriately prior to beginning a review. This is an important, and often overlooked, part of the review process.
- Write reviews as you would like to be reviewed.
- While reviewing, keep in mind the two fundamental aspects of a manuscript: the science and the presentation of the science.
- If you do not understand something, do not be afraid to say so in your review.
- Document the journals for which you are a reviewer on your curriculum vitae.

## QUESTIONS TO DISCUSS WITH A MENTOR OR COLLEAGUE

1. What are my areas of expertise? What topics am I qualified to referee? What journals should I review for?
2. Can I, as an early career psychiatrist, review a manuscript with you, my mentor?
3. How does one balance the critic and the teacher in the review process?
4. When is it okay to say no to a review offer?

## REFERENCES

Black N, van Rooyen S, Godlee F, et al: What makes a good reviewer and a good review for a general medical journal? JAMA 280:231–233, 1998

Bordage G, Caelleigh AS: How to read "review criteria for research manuscripts." Acad Med 76:909–910, 2001

Burnham JC: The evolution of editorial peer review. JAMA 263:1323–1329, 1990

Crandall SJ, Caelleigh AS, Steinecke A: Reference to the literature and documentation. Acad Med 76:925–927, 2001

Crandall SJ, McGaghie WC: Discussion and conclusion: interpretation. Acad Med 76:942–944, 2001

Evans AT, McNutt RA, Fletcher SW, et al: The characteristics of peer reviewers who produce good-quality reviews. J Gen Intern Med 8: 422–428, 1993

Goldbeck-Wood S: What makes a good reviewer of manuscripts? (editorial). BMJ 316:86, 1998

Hoppin FG: How I review an original scientific article. Am J Respir Crit Care Med 166:1019–1023, 2002

McGaghie WC, Bordage G, Shea JA: Problem statement, conceptual framework, and research question. Acad Med 76:923–924, 2001

Pangaro L, McGaghie WC: Scientific conduct. Acad Med 76:950–951, 2001

Regehr G: Presentation of results. Acad Med 76:940–942, 2001

Roberts LW: On the centrality of peer review. Acad Psychiatry 26:221–222, 2002

Roberts LW, Coverdale J, Edenharder K, et al: How to review a manuscript: a "down-to-earth" approach. Acad Psychiatry 28:81–87, 2004:

Steinecke A, Shea JA: Review form. Acad Med 76:916–918, 2001

# Approaching Your First Grant Application and the Grant Review Process

Michele T. Pato, M.D.

Carlos N. Pato, M.D.

Nothing replaces a good idea. The first step in writing any grant, whether it be your first or your last, is starting with a good idea that can be formulated into a researchable question. Although this may seem to be a simple task, it often becomes the tragic flaw in a grant proposal when it is not done. Too often the investigator does not defend the scientific merit, the significance, or what some have called the "So what?" factor behind the grant proposal (Hulley et al. 2001; Pato 1999). This chapter will outline the general principles of grant writing that you can adapt to the specific types of grant applications you may be submitting.

## BACKGROUND

Hulley and colleagues (2001) propose the use of the FINER criteria in assessing the characteristics of a good research question. That is, the question should be Feasible, Interesting, Novel, Ethical, and Relevant. Beyond this, the critical aspect of beginning the grant application is turning this research question into one or more testable hypotheses that can be completed in the time requested in the grant application. Additionally, the question should flow through all parts of the proposal and be clear.

## GETTING PREPARED

### Outline

This is a tool that you are writing for yourself. A two- to three-page outline should state the question you are trying to answer, identify the significance of the work, and briefly map out the research design. Use the outline to define those things you will control or manipulate (*predictor* or *independent variables*) and those things you will measure (*outcome* or *dependent variables*). As you map out the study design, you should consider the specific hypotheses you will be testing, the analytic methods you will have to employ to test them, the statistical power you wish to achieve, and the sample size you will need in order to do it. This outline will help you to set the direction and goals for writing your proposal. It will help you decide where and to whom you need to turn to get information before you begin to write.

### The Questions to Ask

- What background articles must you read to fit your work into the broader context of what has already been done on that topic and to defend its scientific merit?
- What mentors and collaborators, at your institution or elsewhere, might you need on the project, both to help you learn what you don't know and provide their expertise?
- What analytic or statistical expertise should you solicit to help you structure and analyze the studies you plan and the data you gather?
- What preliminary studies must you do to defend the FINER points and to have pilot information on the question you propose?

Furthermore, as you flesh out your outline, you will find that you have already started to write the various components of your proposal (see Table 23–1 and Appendix 23–A). You can see that the questions you pose will help you in writing the abstract and specific aims of the proposal. The significance (see item 7b in Table 23–1) will be critical to writing the background as well as setting your plan for the preliminary studies you will do and report on. The research plan will expand into the methods you will employ.

## THE CONTENT OF THE PROPOSAL

The *abstract* appears first but should be written last. It is a brief presentation of the question, why you are asking it, and how you are going to try to an-

**TABLE 23–1.** Elements of a grant proposal

1. Face page (with necessary signatures)
2. Abstract
3. Table of contents
4. Budget and budget justification
5. Curriculum vitae or biosketch
6. Resources, equipment, and physical facilities
7. Research plan
   a. Specific aims
   b. Background and significance
   c. Preliminary studies/work accomplished to date
   d. Research design including project calendar[a]
8. Ethical considerations
9. References
10. Consultants and letters of collaboration
11. Appendices

[a]In a career development award (K award), the research plan should also include a career development plan, which should have its own calendar for completion.
*Source.* Adapted from PHS 398.

swer it. It is critically important to reviewers that it be well written, concise, integrated, and interesting. The *specific aims* clearly spell out the questions and the testable hypotheses. The *background* is where you lay the foundation for the proposal you are writing. It should clearly state what is known in this area and the relevance of your specific question. The *work accomplished* section presents the work you have done to date with respect to the topic of the proposal at hand. The *research plan* is the structure and body of your proposal. Its purpose is to show the reviewer that you understand the methods and know what it will take to actually do the work; it should also include the timeline for your project (project calendar). *Appendices* can be included but do not have to count in the usual 25-page limit that is the body of the grant. Appendices may be copies of articles that you have published as part of your background or preliminary work, which you will have space to refer to only briefly in the body of the grant. Appendices may also include previously published rating scales that you might be using, but usually only those that may not be familiar to the average reader. *Consultants* and collaborators are critical to the success of any proposal—few investigators will be able to provide all of the expertise needed for a project. You, as the *principal investigator,* are building a team of experts to do the work. Your co-investigators are from your own institution, while outside experts are consultants or collaborators. For a new investigator, the experience another investigator brings to the table can be critical.

*Ethical considerations* (human subjects or animal protection) is a critical section and should be considered before you begin writing your proposal. The issues of ethical treatment of research subjects will help to determine whether the research project should even be pursued. For your first proposal, go to a senior consultant, possibly from the institutional review board, and discuss your proposal. The fundamental constructs of the ethical consideration are the risks of the research and the potential benefits from the outcomes. For human research, the process of informed consent is critical. In addition, investigators are under increased scrutiny, appropriately, and must disclose potential conflicts of interest at the federal, state, and county levels. Be aware of such requirements from your granting agency.

## Budget

Your grant application is a tool for asking for financial support to do your research project. As you get swept up in the process of writing your first proposal, it is easy to lose sight of this main objective. It is critical to start the process early of defining the costs of doing the proposed work. The process of defining costs can affect what funding source you apply to or even what project you can really do. Ideally, this is an iterative process in which the funding constraints help define the scope of the work—you cannot do it all up front or wait and do it all at the end.

The *budget* section of your proposal details and justifies how you will spend the funds granted to you. The resources that will be provided by your institution or any collaborating institutions should to be spelled out and are part of the justification for an agency funding your project. Pay special attention to the budget pages and take the necessary time to fill them out. *Do not wait* until the grant is complete or within a few days of its due date to go to your grants management office and ask for help doing the budget. Many institutions, through their sponsored projects office, usually require a 2–3 week turnaround period to make the various calculations and get the necessary signatures for approval. In addition, they may help inform you about what things will cost, particularly with regard to fringe costs (e.g., benefits), and this may affect the overall research plan. Most proposals have some sort of funding cap, especially those that are often pursued by first-time grant recipients. Therefore, you may need to curtail your research plan once you have a better idea of the actual costs of the personnel, equipment, and fringe costs to the university.

## Getting the Proposal Done

Many beginning investigators underestimate the logistical coordination it takes to start, maintain, and complete a grant submission. We suggest a timeline of at least 12 months to contact the granting agency for information, formulate the research question, collect background information, meet with collaborators, meet with biostatisticians, pull the grant together, and get everything formatted for the grant agency (Table 23–2). The Internet is an important resource for obtaining information about grants as well as grant preparation. Most federal granting agencies, as well as private funding agencies, have Web sites where you can read about requests for applications (RFAs) or find out about specific mechanisms for submitting investigator-initiated grants. An RFA stipulates what areas or topics the grant should cover, whereas in an investigator-initiated grant, the topic and methods of the grant are of your own choosing.

The last step of grant preparation, compiling the grant for submission, can be particularly complex. Careful attention to the details at this stage is important. All necessary components of the grant application must be filled out correctly (Table 23–1) or you risk the proposal being sent back before it is even reviewed. Therefore, you must pay attention to page limits, human subjects protection, and other components that may be uniquely requested by the specific funding agency.

In addition, the overall clarity of the presentation, both in the writing and formatting of the proposal, is very important. A grant application that is difficult to read (e.g., the font is too small or crammed or the margins are too narrow) will distract the reviewer. Errors in grammar and spelling not only reflect poorly on your care and accuracy as a scientist but also make it difficult for the reviewer to focus on the content of your proposal. Always err on the side of saying less with more clarity. Remember the reviewer will be reading a stack of many proposals. You are always better off having yours stand out because it is easy to read. A careful reading of the grant in its final stages by someone with good grammar and spelling skills is essential. Spell check and grammar check will not always catch errors of omission (e.g., "for" and "form") and reversal (e.g., "from" and "form") and other oversights such as missing tables or references. Someone who has not been involved in the actual writing of the proposal and who has only passing familiarity with the subject matter might provide a good simulation of an actual reviewer and help you to identify areas of your proposal that are unclear or don't make smooth transitions. If you do not have someone to read the grant,

---

**TABLE 23–2.**   Timeline for completing your first grant proposal

---

**Over the previous years**   Write and get into press first-author papers based on the area of your grant proposal. Show that you are knowledgeable about the field.

**9 months ahead**   Begin to talk to mentors and potential collaborators about your research idea and potential researchable questions. Consult with a statistician early and often!

**6 months ahead**   Gather and read background literature related to your research question. Find out what has already been done and figure out how you can extend the work in the field. Write your proposal outline. Have someone (e.g., a mentor, advisor, consultant, or collaborator) look over the outline and offer suggestions.

**4 months ahead**   This should be an intensive writing period as you begin to write the pieces of your grant. Start with specific aims and background, move on to the methods, save the abstract for last. As in the last stage, continue to have *several people* look over the pieces of the grant as you write them and offer suggestions. Talk to an institutional review board mentor about ethical considerations.

**2 months ahead**   Show a rough draft to your mentor or advisor for feedback.

**6 weeks ahead**   Bring a rough but complete draft, especially the budget, to the sponsored projects office so they can advise you.

**3–4 weeks ahead**   Submit a nearly completed copy to sponsored projects office to get the signatures you need.

**Last 2 weeks**   Complete all necessary sections. Leave at least 1 week free in your schedule to do this, if possible. Have others read for grammar, spelling, and clarity; make necessary copies and submit (plan on this taking more time than you expect).

---

consider reading it aloud so you can identify awkward sentences and pick out other errors as you turn the visual process of reading into an auditory one.

## THE REVIEW AND DECISION PROCESS

Your proposal will be reviewed by experts in the field, although not necessarily in your area of expertise. This process may take several months from when you initially submit the proposal. Research funding is a competitive process, and many great proposals will need to be revised before they are ultimately funded. Submitting the proposal is the beginning of the process. You should consider your review as not only your score but a guide to how to improve it. In many agencies, fewer than one in five proposals are ultimately funded (for the National Institutes of Health, this would be called the 20th percentile). On the other hand, there are many proposals that were ultimately funded even though they did not do well on their first submission.

A successful investigator is one who is funded for what he or she wants to study, rather than one who gets funding simply to meet academic expectations. Although the academic career track applies both subtle and blatant pressure to be a funded researcher, the most important consideration should be to do a project you believe in.

## SMART STRATEGIES

- Think FINER: **F**easible, **I**nteresting, **N**ovel, **E**thical, **R**elevant.
- Get preliminary data and write first-author papers.
- Work with mentors and advisors; get to know local and distant resources.
- Select an institute or funding agency and type of grant to write.
- Use successful grants as models.
- Write, revise, write, revise, write, revise...
- Have mentors and advisors review the proposal.
- Polish and catch errors in the proposal before making copies to submit.
- Maintain contact with program officers.
- Plan to revise and resubmit your proposal.

## QUESTIONS TO DISCUSS WITH A MENTOR OR COLLEAGUE

1. What institute or funding agency might be interested in funding my grant idea? How might I modify the idea to make it more attractive to the agency or institute?
2. What is a reasonable timetable to complete the grant (given my other commitments and the commitments of my mentor or supervisor)?
3. Does the work proposed in the grant have a good chance of being completed in the time allotted (3–5 years)?
4. Is the research plan clearly articulated in the grant, and does it have enough flexibility to be completed if things change?
5. Have I provided enough background in the grant for reviewers without specific expertise to understand what is being proposed and its scientific merit?

# REFERENCES

Hulley SB, Cummings SR, Browner WS, et al: Designing Clinical Research, 2nd Edition. Philadelphia, PA, Lippincott William and Wilkins, 2001

Pato MT: Generating and implementing research ideas, in Handbook of Psychiatric Education and Faculty Development. Edited by Kay J, Silberman E, Pessar L. Washington, DC, American Psychiatric Press, 1999, pp 181–194

# ADDITIONAL RESOURCES

National Institutes of Health: Grants and funding opportunities. Available at: http://grants1.nih.gov/grants/. Accessed March 8, 2005.

National Institutes of Health: Inside the NIH grant review process: a video on peer review at NIH. Available at: http://www.csr.nih.gov/Video/Video_print.asp. Accessed March 8, 2005.

Walders N, Tanielian T, Pincus HA: Getting funding for research, in Handbook of Psychiatric Education and Faculty Development. Edited by Kay J, Silberman E, Pessar L. Washington, DC, American Psychiatric Press, 1999, pp 195–213

# APPENDIX 23–A

## SAMPLE BIOSKETCH

Principal Investigator/Program Director (Last, First, Middle):  PI Name

### BIOGRAPHICAL SKETCH

Provide the following information for the key personnel and other significant contributors in the order listed on Form Page 2.
Follow this format for each person. **DO NOT EXCEED FOUR PAGES.**

| NAME | POSITION TITLE |
|---|---|
| Carlucci, Joseph Louis | Professor of Microbiology |
| eRA COMMONS USER NAME | |
| Carluccij | |

EDUCATION/TRAINING *(Begin with baccalaureate or other initial professional education, such as nursing, and include postdoctoral training.)*

| INSTITUTION AND LOCATION | DEGREE *(if applicable)* | YEAR(s) | FIELD OF STUDY |
|---|---|---|---|
| Stanford University | Ph.D. | 1964 | Infectious Diseases |
| Harvard Medical School | M.D. | 1972 | Medicine/Parasitology |

## A. Positions and Honors.

### Positions and Employment
| | |
|---|---|
| 1969-1971 | Medical Residency, Internal Medicine, Harvard Medical School |
| 1971-1973 | EIS Officer, Hospital Infection Section, Bacterial Diseases Branch, CDC, Atlanta, GA |
| 1973-1974 | Instructor and Fellow in Medicine, Hematology, Massachusetts General Hospital, Boston, MA |
| 1974-1975 | Instructor in Infectious Diseases, Massachusetts General Hospital, Boston, MA |
| 1978- | Senior Associate in Infectious Diseases, Children's Hospital, Boston, MA |
| 1978-1984 | Assistant Professor of Pediatrics, Harvard Medical School |
| 1985-1998 | Chief, Hemostasis Laboratory, Children's Hospital, Boston, MA |
| 1993- | Professor of Pediatrics, Harvard Medical School, Boston, MA |
| 1998- | Professor, Dept. of Infectious Diseases, Harvard School of Public Health |

### Other Experience and Professional Memberships
| | |
|---|---|
| 1972-1973 | Acting Chief, National Mucosal Infections Study |
| 1975-2000 | Director of Infectious Diseases Laboratory |
| 1975-present | Hospital Epidemiologist (Medical Director Infection Control 2000-present), Children's Hospital, Boston |
| 1981-1982 | President, Society of Hospital Epidemiologists of America |
| 1988 | Member, Society for Pediatric Research |
| 1989-present | Medical Director Quality Assurance, Children's Hospital, Boston, MA |
| 1991-1993 | Director, American Society for Microbiology, Division F |
| 1991-1997 | Hospital Infection Control Practices Advisory Committee, Centers for Disease Control |
| 1998-present | Vice-Chair for Health Outcomes, Dept. of Medicine, Children's Hospital |
| 1998-2001 | Steering Committee, NACHRI/CDC Pediatric Prevention Network |

### Honors
| | |
|---|---|
| 1982 | SERC Advanced Research Scholarship, Infectious Disease Society of America |
| 2001 | Anthony Steinway Award for Excellence in Teaching (Children's Hospital) |

## B. Selected peer-reviewed publications (in chronological order).

(Publications selected from 133 peer-reviewed publications)

1. Luciani JM, Casper J, Goodman BF, Shaw CM, Carlucci JL. Prevention of respiratory virus infections through compliance with frequent hand-washing routines. N Engl J Med 1988 ;318:389-394.

2. Gussmann J, Pratt R, Sideway DG, Sinclair JM, Emmerson MF, Carlucci JL. Coagulase-negative staphylococcal bacteremia in the changing neonatal intensive care unit population. Is there an epidemic? JAMA. 1988;158:1548-1552.

3. Gussmann J, Carlucci JL, McGovern JE, Jr., Methodologic issues in nursing home epidemiology. Rev Infect Dis 1989;11:1119-1141.

4. Gussmann J, Emmerson MF, Smyth NE, Platt RI, Sidebottom DG, Carlucci JL. Early hospital release and antibiotic usage with nosocomial staphylococcal bacteremia in two neonatal intensive care unit populations. Amer J Dis Child 1991;149:325-339.

5. Murphy JA, Black RW, Schroeder LC, Weissman ST, Gussman JM, Carlucci JL, Short CJ. Quality of care for children with asthma: the role of social factors and practice setting. Pediatrics 1996;98:379-84.

6. Gussmann J, Carlucci JL, McGovern JE, Jr. Incidence of Staphylococcus epidermidis catheter-related bacteremia by infusions. J Infect Dis 1996;172:320-4.

7. Carlucci JL, Huskins WC. Control of nosocomial antimicrobial-resistant bacteria A strategic priority for hospitals worldwide. Clin Infect Dis 1997;S139-S145.

8. Corning WC, Saylor BM, O'Steen C, Gulapagos L, O'Reilly EJ, Carlucci JL. Hospital infection prevention and control: A model for improving the quality of hospital care in low income countries. Infect Control Hosp Epi. 1999;13:123-35.

9. Handler CJ, Marriott B, Clearwater PT, Carlucci JL. Quality of care at a children's hospital: the child's perspective. Arch Pediatr Adolesc Med. 1999;143:1120-7.

10. McKinney D, Poulet KL, Wong Y, Murphy V, Ulright M, Dorling G, Long JC, Carlucci JL, Piper GB. Protective vaccine for Staphylococcus aureus. Science 1999;214:1421-7.

11. Gulazzii L, Kispert ZT, Carlucci JL, Corning WC. Risk-adjusted mortality rates in surgery: a model for outcome measurement in hospitals developing new quality improvement programs. J Hosp Infect 2000;24:33-42.

12. Huebner J, Qui A, Krueger WA, Carlucci JL, Pier GB. Prophylactic and therapeutic efficacy of antibodies to a capsular polysaccharide shared among vancomycin-sensitive and resistant enterococci. Infect Inmmun 2000; 68:4631-6.

13. Levitan O, Sissy RB, Kenney J, Buchwald E, Maccharone AB, Carlucci JL. Enhancement of neonatal innate defense: Effects of adding an recombinant fragment of bactericidal protein on growth and tumor necrosis factor-inducing activity of gram-positive bacteria tested in vivo. Immun 2000;38:3120-25.

14. Garletti JS, Harrison MC, Collin PA, Miller CD, Otter D, Shaker C, Wren M, Carlucci JL, Makato DG. A randomized trial comparing iodine to a alcohol impregnated dressing for prevention of catheter infections in neonates. Pediatrics. 2001;127:1461-6.

15. Corning WC, Barillo K, Festival MR, Lingonberry S, Lumbar P, Peters A, Pursons M, Carlucci JL, Tella JE. A national survey of practice variation in the use of antibiotic prophylaxis in heart surgery. J Hosp Infect. 2001;33:121-5.

16. Hoboken S, Peterson D, Graveldy L, Carlucci JL. Compliance with hand hygiene practice in pediatric intensive care. Pediatric Crit Care Med. 2001;12:211-214.

17. Hasker S, Pittoui D, Gray L, Zaruccii A, Potter G, Seemore MH, Carlucci JL. Interventional study to evaluate the impact of an antibiotic-infused hand gel in improving hand hygiene compliance. Pediatr Infect Dis J. Accepted for publication.

18. Lander C, Summers R, Murray S, Hummer CJ, Carlucci JL. Pediatrics: Is hospital food more nutritional than mom's cooking? Pediatrics 2001;11: 140-145.

## C. Research Support

<u>Ongoing Research Support</u>
R01 HS35793  Carlucci (PI)                    9/01/99-8/30/04
AHRQ
Reducing Antimicrobial Resistance in Low-Income Communities: A Randomized Trial.

This study is a randomized trial of interventions to reduce antimicrobial usage and resistance in low-income communities.
Role: PI

2 R01 AI12345-05   Carlucci (PI)             4/01/01-3/31/06
NIH/NIAID
Bacteriology and Mycology Study of ICU Patients at Risk for Antimicrobial Resistant Bacterial Infections.
The study will perform clinical trials of interventions to reduce antimicrobial resistant infections.
Role: PI

R01- AI24680-04  Peterson (PI)             3/01/01-2/28/06
NIH/NIAID
Virulence and Immunity to Staphylococci.
This study investigates the production of polysaccharide by *Staphylococcus aureus* and its role in virulence as measured in animal models of infection and its ability to function as a target for protective antibody.
Role: Paid consultant.

2 R01 HL 00000-13 Anderson (PI)            3/01/01-2/28/06
NIH/NHLBI
Chloride and Sodium Transport in Airway Epithelial Cells
The major goals of this project are to define the biochemistry of chloride and sodium transport in airway epithelial cells and clone the gene(s) involved in transport.
Role: Co-Investigator

5 R01 HL 00000-07 Baker (PI)              4/1/01 – 3/31/04
NIH/NHLBI
Ion Transport in Lungs
The major goal of this project is to study chloride and sodium transport in normal and diseased lungs.
Role: Co-Investigator

1 R01 AI12826-01   Hoffman (PI)            9/28/01-9/27/03
NIH/NIAID
Intermountain Child Health Services Research Consortium
This consortium will seek to build pediatric health services research capacity and training in the Intermountain Region.
Role: Co-Investigator

## <u>Completed Research Support</u>

5 RO1 AI10011-05 Herman (PI)             12/01/00 – 11/30/04
NIH/NIAID
Evaluating Quality Improvement Strategies (EQUIS)
The goal of this study was to evaluate quality improvement and collaborative learning to improve asthma care in office-based pediatrics.
Role: Co-Investigator

5 R01 AI098765 Spielman (PI)            7/01/99 -6/30/04
NIH/NIAID
Epidemiology of Emerging Infections #1 T32 AI07654
The goal of this project was to study emerging infections in high risk populations who are treated in emergency room situations.
Role: Co-Investigator

*Source.*   http://grants2nih.gov/grants/funding/phs398/biosketchsample.pdf

# Approaching Research, Evaluation, and Continuous Quality Improvement Projects

Donald M. Hilty, M.D.

Martin H. Leamon, M.D.

Laura Weiss Roberts, M.D., M.A.

Data gathering is an important part of many different academic activities. After we give a lecture, we receive written feedback from learners; when we review patient charts for administrative and quality assurance purposes, we gather information (sometimes very sensitive information) from these "primary sources"; when we study the responses of participants in clinical trials, we collect diverse biological and psychosocial information. Although the aims of these activities differ—they aim, respectively, to improve teaching, ensure appropriate standards of care, and generate new knowledge—they share the common feature of data gathering in an academic environment. Moreover, under some circumstances, because of the special nature of the data we work with, these activities fall under regulatory safeguards. These safeguards are intended to protect the interests and well-being of people we are entrusted to serve through our roles as teachers, clinicians, researchers, and academic administrators.

It is important for the early career faculty member to be aware of issues that affect his or her everyday data-gathering activities. National guidelines govern certain activities (e.g., involvement of human subjects, release of clinical information) in "silos"—but there are gaps and overlaps between different domains of activity for an academic faculty member. Often faculty members are not sure into which silo (or silos) a given project fits. This chapter will review a variety of potential activities that elucidate boundaries between and within different data-gathering activities. Attention to these issues will help an early career faculty member be sure that he or she complies with local, state, and federal requirements and that patients' and trainees' rights and interests are honored.

## TYPES OF STUDIES, GUIDELINES, AND AGENCIES

U.S. federal regulation 45 CFR 46.102(d) defines research as "a systematic investigation, including research development, testing and evaluation, designed to develop or contribute to generalizable knowledge" (Public Health Service Act 1985). Interpreting this definition accurately and applying it to one's work correctly are very important. For instance, a faculty member may gather data from her students regarding a new seminar or educational experience *without* any formal monitoring by the institutional review board (IRB), so long as the data are collected solely for the purpose of improving the educational activity. Similarly, data may be collected regarding clinical care activities *without* any formal oversight, so long as the data are collected solely for the purpose of assuring appropriate clinical care and "doing business" (e.g., billing and collections). However, if the faculty member's intent changes at any point in the process—from "quality improvement" or "quality assurance" to scholarly or specific research goals—then IRB approval and oversight may be necessary. A specific example would be a teacher gathering feedback on a community-based learning experience. When the faculty member forms the impression that the experience is inspiring many students to go into psychiatry, and then wants to reexamine the data or collect new data with the intent of presenting the findings at a professional meeting or in a journal publication, then the IRB should be formally involved (e.g., to assess whether the project meets criteria for exemption, or to approve the project).

All science activities are subject to university, state, and federal guidelines. Research involving animals is very vigorously protected by professional codes and federal rules (Gluck et al. 2002). These include animal welfare regulations, which require that all federally funded research facilities using animals establish an Institutional Animal Care and Use Committee (IACUC). Helpful resources for learning more about animal research can be found at http://ehs.ucdavis.edu/animal/index.cfm, and a second Web site has a step-by-step tutorial at http://tutorials.rgs.uci.edu.

Research involving the participation of living human volunteers is a carefully regulated, vigilantly monitored endeavor and has met with considerable controversy over the years (Roberts and Roberts 1999). Very prestigious university programs have been halted and individual investigators have been suspended because of systematic failures in implementing appropriate safeguards. The Federal Office of Human Research Protection oversees programs in the United States through local offices of vice-chancellors of research and institutional review boards—independently of deans of colleges—to avoid potential institutional conflict of interest.

Certain types of research are generally exempt from the 45 CFR 46 regulations, as detailed in 45 CFR 46.101(b). These include 1) "Research conducted in established or commonly accepted educational settings, involving normal educational practices…;" 2) "Research involving the use of educational tests…, survey procedures, interview procedures or observation of public behavior, unless…[individual] human subjects can be identified…;" 3) "Research involving …existing data…or …specimens, if these sources are publicly available or if …subjects cannot be identified, directly or [indirectly]….;" and 4) "Taste and food quality evaluation and consumer acceptance studies…."

It should be noted, however, that federal authorities retain final judgment as to whether or not a specific research activity is exempt, and federal law does not exempt an investigator from state or local regulations that may apply.

Computer-based tutorials on key issues for investigators, staff, and IRB members are available through federal (e.g., http://ohsr.od.nih.gov/cbt/) and university (e.g., http://tutorials.rgs.uci.edu) Web sites. The latter site has programs on the following topics:

- Human research issues (e.g., informed consent, confidentiality, and other issues)
- National Institutes of Health (NIH) Certificate of Confidentiality (i.e., protecting identifiable research information from forced disclosure in any civil, criminal, administrative, legislative, or other proceeding; see http://grants.nih.gov/grants/policy/coc/index.htm)
- Environmental health and safety

- Health Insurance Portability and Accountability Act (HIPAA) (1996) research; this is a specific adaptation to more general databases (e.g., U.S. Department of Health and Human Services, http://www.hhs .gov/ocr/hipaa)
- Use of recombinant DNA

## CONFLICTS OF INTEREST

Another key issue in research is financial disclosure and avoidance of conflicts of interest; these ethically important considerations also fall under regulatory guidelines. *Financial disclosure* pertains to whether or not any of the study personnel might stand to benefit financially from the study depending on the results. *Conflict of interest* pertains to other potential nonfinancial gains—for example, a clinician-researcher might receive a better personnel evaluation if his or her patients, who are the test subjects, improve more than the control subjects treated by a competitive colleague.

The Association of American Medical Colleges (AAMC) released the first report of its Task Force on Conflicts of Interest in Clinical Research, *Protecting Subjects, Preserving Trust, Promoting Progress: Policy and Guidelines for the Oversight of Individual Interests in Research* (Association of American Medical Colleges 2005). The guidelines propose that institutions adopt high standards for the reporting, review, and disclosure of researchers' financial interests in federally funded and privately sponsored human subjects research. The key focus of the report is the recommendation that academic institutions presume that a "financially interested individual"—defined in the report as any researcher holding a significant financial interest in human subject research—share those issues with the appropriate IRB and an evaluation be made regarding disclosure to subjects. The guidelines underscore the necessity of disclosing financial interests in human subjects research in publications and presentations. New NIH guidelines pertaining to research-related conflicts of interest were released in February 2005.

Some data-gathering activities are not intended as research per se; that is, the information is not collected with the intent of contributing to new knowledge. In such situations, an early career faculty member may be unclear about what falls under whose administrative purview. For instance, a hospital's patient care ethics committee may offer opinions on controversial studies that have already been approved by the medical school's IRB. Similarly, a physician may collect patient data on one day in the context of a quality assurance effort and the very next day collect patient data in a similar way for a research project. The two activities seem alike, but they fall into different regulatory categories. (This is naturally very confusing!) Recent changes associated with HIPAA regulations make this set of issues even more complex (http://www.hhs.gov/ocr/hipaa). It is important to be sure that the activity you've undertaken is done with the correct approval and administrative supports or protections.

There are special compliance issues pertaining to the overlaps and distinctions in quality assurance (or continuous quality improvement) activities and human research. Hospital programs are also regulated by the Joint Commission on Accreditation of Healthcare Organizations (JCAHO) and the National Committee for Quality Assurance (NCQA) with regard to quality improvement and human subject protection programs. The new organization Partnership for Human Research Protection, Inc. (PHRP) has issued draft accreditation standards that are available for public comment (http://www.jcaho.org).

## PROBLEMS AND SOLUTIONS REGARDING STUDIES AND PROJECTS

The following three cases illustrate the complexities encountered in performing what appear to be routine data-gathering activities in one's faculty role.

### Case Example 1

> The residency training director announces his intention to study concept mapping (i.e., how learners make connections between ideas and concepts) in residents. He announces that residents do not have to participate but that it would help the training program if they were to do so. The training director will lead the project and several sessions with residents who attend. Residents may earn $175 from department funds to participate for 4 hours.

Potential problems:

- The training director has a dual role as both a researcher and a training director and supervisor in this scenario. This introduces a potential set of conflicting interests and adds significantly greater ethical complexity to the situation. Some residents may feel obligated to participate, despite reassurances that they do not have to, because the training director will know who did and who did not participate. Furthermore, as both learners in the program and research participants, the residents may feel that they are in a double-jeopardy situation, in which their concept maps will be used both for learner evaluation and as data.

- The level of participant compensation has to be evaluated to see whether it is coercive.

Potential solutions:

- Separate the roles of training director and researcher by having another faculty member conduct the study or, alternatively, having the training director-researcher conduct the work at another program or institution in a collaborative fashion.
- Simply implement concept mapping as a required form of evaluation for all residents. Concept mapping has been used in a number of programs and could be seen as normal educational practice. No money would be offered. Evaluation of concept mapping could be conducted internally, but if the decision was made to disseminate the results in order to contribute to generalizable knowledge, strict attention would need to be paid to resident anonymity. At that point, IRB review of a study involving existing data of educational evaluations would be appropriate.

Who (at a minimum) reviews the proposal?

- The department
- The university IRB, because it involves human participants

Principles and guidelines to remember:

- Anonymity is important, so as to avoid conflicts of interest.
- "Authority" is subject to (mis)perceptions by trainees.
- The IRB has the final say on whether this project can be conducted. Moreover, the IRB may not give permission in light of the participants' dual roles, potential coercion, and privacy-related concerns, even though this is a minimal-risk educational study.

## Case Example 2

A clinical researcher and a child psychiatrist decide to participate in an outpatient randomized, controlled trial of placebo versus study medication for adolescents with bipolar disorder. The IRB has an adult psychiatrist member, but she feels a little uncomfortable evaluating a proposal with a focus beyond her scope of practice.

Potential problems and solutions:

- Are placebo-controlled trials acceptable in children, adolescents, and adults?

- This depends on the disorder, standard of care, risk, inclusion criteria (e.g., suicidal ideation in adolescent outpatients may preclude enrollment), local precedents, and review criteria.
- At the very least, prospective reviews by the IRB, a child psychiatrist, and relevant members of the community are in order.

- If a placebo-controlled trial in children or adolescents is done, what safeguards, in addition to the usual, may be necessary?

  - Careful collaboration with parents
  - Monitoring one to two times a week for worsening of depression or dangerous side effects
  - Psychotherapy, which may be the standard of care (e.g., cognitive-behavioral therapy)

Who (at a minimum) reviews the proposal?

- The department
- The university IRB
- A mood disorder psychiatrist or child psychiatrist
- A community organization (e.g., National Alliance for the Mentally Ill)

Principles and guidelines to remember:

- Seek help from a variety of others in the department, university, and community on controversial projects.
- Building in appropriate safeguards up front will protect the patient, family, investigator, department, and university.

## Case Example 3

A faculty member decides to do a needs assessment for cultural psychiatric consultation services at 20 rural primary care sites using telepsychiatry. She plans to fax the survey to rural coordinators and physicians to collect information about clinic patterns and needs (but not about individual patients). The survey covers sociodemographics of patients, their language skills, and use of interpreters (formal or family).

Potential problems:

- It is not clear whether this is just an attempt to improve services, as part of continuous quality improvement, or to conduct research.

  - This depends on the true intent of the project, as well as whether collecting this information would be a standard part of clinical service administration.

- The faculty did not run the project through the department, because the service is outside its administrative boundary, or the Center for Health and Technology, which oversees telemedicine.

Potential solutions:

- If the intent of the study remains unclear, speak with the IRB; It may feel that this is beyond the scope of routine services and may request data for an exemption.
- The investigator may have benefited from the input of the Center for Health and Technology; she needs its buy-in in case questions or issues arise. In addition, the Center needs to know what goes on within its borders.
- The Center approves the survey, offers suggestions, adds a few questions for its own purpose, and helps fax it.

Who (at a minimum) reviews the proposal?

- The department
- The university IRB
- Possibly the university or Clinic Legal Department (e.g., to verify HIPAA compliance measures)
- The center (or clinic) of project origin

Principles and guidelines to remember:

- Seek advice from administrators and the IRB when it may not be clear under whose jurisdiction a project falls.
- Recall that the project will require approval by the IRB if ever the project intent changes from clinical service enhancement to the goal of contributing to generalizable knowledge, for example, through eventual publication.

## CONCLUSIONS

In sum, the daily activities of an academic faculty member commonly involve collecting information. Data gathering falls under different regulatory requirements depending on the circumstances, and the ethical, compliance, and legal issues that accompany data gathering are extremely important. Early career faculty members should become familiar with different regulations and resources related to these activities and always seek consultation from knowledgeable colleagues, institutional leaders, and national experts when difficult questions arise.

## SMART STRATEGIES

- Remember that anonymity may be important when trainees are participating in research.
- Avoid, declare, or resolve conflicts of interest.
- Be aware that authority is subject to (mis)perceptions by trainees, subjects, and others.
- Gain consent for contact and release of information, particularly mental health information.
- Conduct chart reviews anonymously and with identities hidden and information securely locked.
- Seek help from a variety of others in the department, university, and community on controversial projects.
- Protect the patient, family, investigator, department, and university by using safeguards.
- Seek advice from administrators and the IRB to clarify whether a project constitutes continued quality improvement or research.
- Recall that almost always, approval by the IRB is needed for eventual publication.
- Guidelines are continually changing—stay updated!

## QUESTIONS TO DISCUSS WITH A MENTOR OR COLLEAGUE

1. How might systematic data gathering enhance my everyday academic activities?
2. What data-gathering activities am I doing, and what regulatory safeguards may be applicable to these activities?
3. What institutional resources exist to help with data-gathering efforts?

## REFERENCES

Association of American Medical Colleges: Conflict of Interest in Clinical Research. 2005. Available at: http://www.aamc.org/coitf.

Gluck JP, DiPasquale T, Orlans FB (eds): Applied Ethics in Animal Research: Philosophy, Regulation, and Laboratory Applications. Purdue, IN, Purdue University Press, 2002

Health Information Portability and Accountability Act of 1996. Regulations available at: http://www.hhs/ocr/hipaa.

Public Health Service Act, amended by the Health Research Extension Act of 1985. Title 45 Code of Regulations, Part 46, Protection of Human Subjects. Available at: http://www.hhs.gov/ohrp/humansubjects/guidance/statute .htm.

Roberts LW, Roberts B: Psychiatric research ethics: an overview of evolving guidelines and current ethical dilemmas in the study of mental illness. Biol Psychiatry 46:1025–1038, 1999

## ADDITIONAL RESOURCES

Jonsen AR, Siegler M, Winslade WJ: Clinical Ethics: A Practical Approach to Ethical Decisions in Clinical Medicine, 2nd Edition. New York, Macmillan, 1986

Penslar RL: Human subject protections: basic IRB review [U.S. Department of Health and Human Services Web site]. Available at: http://www.hhs.gov/ohrp/irb/irb_chapter3.htm. Accessed March 8, 2005.

# PART VI

# Continuing to Grow Professionally...

# CHAPTER 25

# Approaching Certification and Maintenance of Certification

Stephen Scheiber, M.D.

Laura Weiss Roberts, M.D., M.A.

Donald M. Hilty, M.D.

Board certification is among the most important milestones in a psychiatrist's professional life. It is a rigorous process that serves to consolidate years of learning and to determine and affirm one's competence as a specialist physician. The initial certification examination entails knowledge-based and performance-based components, and this rigorous evaluative process may be anxiety provoking for many early career psychiatrists. Recertification involves only knowledge-based testing and verifying the candidate's up-to-date knowledge of the field. It is important to prepare carefully for this sequence of examinations.

Certification and recertification may be seen positively as a formal means of lifelong learning. Just as runners need to maintain fitness with practice, new techniques, and input from others, we seek educational fitness by maintaining our expertise in clinical medicine and other endeavors. This chapter seeks to help early career academic psychiatrists develop a structured, constructive approach to professional board certification. The aim is to provide background on board certification by the American Board of Psychiatry and Neurology (ABPN), to offer information about the process of obtaining certification and recertification in psychiatry, and to help academically committed early career psychiatrists to see this process as a valuable part of a lifelong endeavor to learn and grow professionally.

## BACKGROUND AND RELEVANCE FOR ACADEMIC PSYCHIATRY

The ABPN was formed in 1934 and began issuing certificates in 1935. It is one of the 24 member boards of the American Board of Medical Specialties (ABMS), the organization that develops policies for certification and maintenance of certification. The ABPN and its diplomats represent the fields of psychiatry and neurology within the broader profession of medicine.

The ABPN issues primary certificates in psychiatry and neurology, with special qualification in child neurology. In addition, psychiatrists may obtain subspecialty certification in addiction psychiatry, child and adolescent psychiatry, clinical neurophysiology, geriatric psychiatry, forensic psychiatry, pain medicine, and, beginning in 2005, psychosomatic medicine. Neurologists and child neurologists may seek subspecialty certification in clinical neurophysiology, neurodevelopment disabilities (child neurologists), pain medicine, and vascular neurology. The ABPN has submitted an application for a certificate in neuromuscular medicine for neurologists to the ABMS. In addition, a certificate in sleep medicine along with the American Board of Internal Medicine and the American Board of Pediatrics has been approved, and an examination should be in place no earlier than 2007. This will be available to both psychiatrists and neurologists.

The primary purpose of certification and maintenance of certification is to protect the public. It is also a way for specialists to demonstrate to their peers and to institutions and organizations that they meet essential standards of the field. The certification examinations, which had previously been given in a paper-and-pencil format, are now administered by computer.

There are a number of texts that may be valuable in preparing for the examinations (see Additional Resources in this chapter). The ABPN has also published information on core competencies in psychiatry (available at: http://www.abpn.com/geninfo/competencies.html); over time, individuals sitting for ABPN examinations will demonstrate their mastery of these core competencies.

Most academic institutions require faculty members to become board certified within a reasonable length of time after graduation from an Accreditation Council for Graduate Medical Education (ACGME)–accredited residency program. Faculty members identified as subspecialists in ABMS-approved subspecialties, particularly those who are responsible for teaching and research in those areas, are usually also expected to obtain subspecialty certification.

Academic psychiatrists are in a favorable position to prepare for their certification examinations. They have excellent access to knowl-edgeable colleagues (many of whom may serve as examiners for the ABPN), textbooks, recent literature, and teaching opportunities that help to strengthen one's knowledge and skills set. There are many board review courses offered by both academic departments and independent vendors. These tend to be expensive, and they vary in utility. In general, these courses should not be necessary for academic psychiatrists to be effective in preparing for the certification process.

Certification in psychiatry is a two-step process: a multiple-choice examination (Part I) that must be passed to sit for the oral examination (Part II). Each of these will now be described.

## APPROACHING THE PART I EXAMINATION

It is prudent for faculty members to sit for examination as soon after res-idency as is possible. To do this, residents in their PGY4 year should sub-mit a completed application along with the application fee to the ABPN by the February 1 deadline. On completion of the residency in June, training directors must submit evidence to the ABPN of the trainee's satisfactory completion of the residency. Once an application is ac-cepted, candidates will receive a content outline describing what topics will be covered on the examination. The psychiatry component of the Part I examination for 2005 includes 1) development through the life cycle, 6%; 2) neurosciences, 10%; 3) behavioral and social sciences, 5%; 4) epidemiology and public policy, 5%; 5) diagnostic procedures, 9%; 6) psychiatric disorders, 30%; 7) treatment of psychiatric disorders, 30%; and 8) special topics (e.g., suicide, ethics), 5%. The neurology component includes 1) basic science aspects of neurologic disorders, 20%; 2) incidence/risk of neurologic disorders, 5%; 3) diagnostic procedures related to neurologic disorders, 20%; 4) clinical evaluation of neurologic disorders/syndromes, 35%; and 5) management and treatment of neurologic disorders, 20%. Well-established knowledge is emphasized on the examination. Both components must be passed to pass the examination.

Candidates may request to take the Part I examination at one of the 200 or more Pearson VUE computer centers in the United States. Re-sponding to the request for a test site and date as soon as Pearson VUE announces the availability maximizes the possibility of getting first choice for both the site and the date.

The key to passing the Part I examination is to study the basic clinical and science materials and to begin this effort long before the actual test (i.e., at least 4–6 months in advance). The best-prepared candidates are those who have absorbed the basic science literature of psychiatry and of neurology and have a grasp of the clinical neurology that is most relevant to the practice of psychiatry. There is a high correlation between performance on the Psychiatry Residents In Training Examination (PRITE) administered by the American College of Psychiatrists and the Part I examination of the ABPN for psychiatry content; there is also a strong correlation between performance on the PRITE and on the Part I for neurology content. Therefore, candidates can use the results of the PRITE to help guide their studies, particularly in identifying those subjects requiring additional attention. In their studies, it is probably wise for candidates to use up-to-date textbooks that contain recent but well-established knowledge, rather than the most recent journal articles containing novel scientific information.

Academic psychiatrists usually know the method of study that works best for them. For example, some individuals do best studying with a small group of colleagues who are planning to sit for the same examination. Other candidates may prefer to study on their own. In either case, it is important to undertake preparation efforts well in advance of the test and to be thorough in one's approach to this high-stakes professional examination. This is especially important for topics that may appear on the test regarding conditions either 1) rare in the general population or 2) rare in the context of one's particular training experiences. This is not a time to wing it.

## MOVING ON TO THE PART II EXAMINATION

After successfully passing the Part I examination, candidates are then eligible for the Part II examination, which is performance based. Because the psychiatry residency review committee requires a clinical evaluation of residents twice during the residency training period, most programs use a mock board format to meet this requirement, and hence residents are exposed to the Part II format.

The current format for the Part II examination is composed of two elements: 1) a live patient interview with a follow-up discussion and 2) a discussion of a videotaped patient interview. These two elements may occur in either order during the actual test situation.

For the live interviews, candidates perform an observed half-hour patient interview that is then followed by a 30-minute presentation and discussion. Examining the patient includes establishing rapport, requires interviewing skill, and places importance on clarification of issues related to patient illness, safety, and clinical care. The presentation includes patient identification, chief complaint, life circumstance, history of present illness, pertinent life history, formal mental status examination, case formulation, differential diagnosis, final working diagnosis, management and treatment plan for the patient, and a statement regarding prognosis. About 10 minutes is devoted to the case presentation, 10 minutes to the case formulation and differential diagnosis, and 10 minutes to discussion of management, treatment, and prognosis.

For the videotape-related portion of the Part II examination, candidates view a videotape of an interview of a patient with mental illness; the interview is conducted by a psychiatrist and is intended to illustrate key issues but may not be a complete diagnostic evaluation. Afterwards, the candidate is evaluated by examiners via a 30-minute discussion of the patient that is similar to the discussion in the live patient interview portion of the exam.

In either format, examiners focus on issues that relate to basic competence and safety. Although no particular model is preferred for assessment and treatment, attending to biological, psychological, and social issues as *specifically* pertinent to the patient is important. Candidates may not bring notes with them into the testing situation, but they may take brief notes during the examination. It is wise to not let the note-taking interfere with establishing rapport with the patient, however.

Anxiety is one of the reasons that candidates are often not at their best during an oral examination. Whereas a candidate approaches Part I by studying, the best investment for the Part II examination is to practice the half-hour examination of the patient followed by a half-hour presentation. One to two practice sessions may be helpful, but it does not hurt to do five or six sessions. Anxiety may be simulated by having a senior examiner present (i.e., department chair) or doing it in front of a group (e.g., 10 students). While this may feel uncomfortable or even embarrassing, psychiatrists on academic faculties often serve or have served as examiners for the Part II examination and can therefore assist their junior colleagues by serving as surrogate examiners. It is important not to let this advantage slip away. This approach may help candidates be more effective in the real test situation.

## MAINTENANCE OF CERTIFICATION

Starting in the early 1990s, the ABPN moved to issuing 10-year, time-limited certificates to candidates who had successfully passed Part I and Part II of the Boards and to candidates who had successfully passed subspecialty certification examinations. Subspecialists must also participate in a maintenance of certification program, again with an examination administered at least every 10 years. For the subspecialties, keeping up with advances in the field through journal articles, textbooks, and attending courses will prepare diplomates for the examinations.

A new initiative has been undertaken to help ensure competence of psychiatrists through maintenance of certification. The program has four components: 1) evidence of an unlimited medical license to indicate professional standing; 2) passing a knowledge-based cognitive examination focused on clinical case material and the practice of general psychiatry; 3) evidence of lifetime learning and self-assessment through continuing medical education (CME) activities (i.e., a yearly average of 30 hours of specialty-specific participation); and 4) assessment of actual psychiatric practice. Of these, the fourth element, involving practice performance assessment, is currently under development. It will be implemented in coming years and will likely be a self-improvement model whereby psychiatrists will compare their practice with evidence-based guidelines and then demonstrate that by doing so, they have improved in their own practice.

Certification and recertification are vital steps in the process of lifelong learning. After the rigorous training of medical school and residency, these further steps may seem unnecessary—it is certainly true that the process of becoming a psychiatrist is immensely time-intensive and requires great dedication and ability. But these periods of intensive learning are also time-limited, and the scientific basis of the field of medicine is growing rapidly. As a consequence, physicians need to sustain and build their knowledge, skills, and expertise over the full course of their careers. CME is one helpful element in lifelong learning, although it places emphasis on content expertise and knowledge rather than other aspects of a specialist physician's professional development (e.g., sophisticated medical decision making, application of novel scientific information to clinical practice). Certification represents a key effort in educational fitness—a disciplined and sustained endeavor to strengthen one's expertise in clinical medicine generally and in psychiatry particularly, as well as to ensure safe and up-to-date clinical practice for society as a whole.

## SMART STRATEGIES

- Do not postpone taking the certification and recertification examinations.
- Prepare early—at least 4–6 months ahead of an examination date.
- Be systematic and organized, paying particular attention to gaps in your experience, understanding, or skills.

- Focus on established knowledge in the field.
- Use the method of study that works best for you (e.g., study group, individual, or both).
- For the knowledge-based examinations, practice on many test-type items such as those on the PRITE.
- For the performance-based examinations, do several practice interviews with follow-up discussion (i.e., mock boards).
- Stretch yourself—practice your interviewing and case presentation skills with a supervisor who will be honest with your performance (to simulate the real test situation, choose someone who is a little bit intimidating).
- Avoid self-defeating study habits.
- View the certification process constructively as a part of lifelong learning and educational fitness.

## QUESTIONS TO DISCUSS WITH A MENTOR OR COLLEAGUE

1. In your experience, what has been a successful strategy for preparing for the Part I exam? For Part II?
2. What are my strengths? What are my areas for improvement in terms of knowledge, verbal presentation skills, and case formulation?
3. What value has board certification brought to your professional development?

## ADDITIONAL RESOURCES

American Board of Psychiatry and Neurology, Inc [ABPN Web site]. Available at: www.abpn.com. Accessed March 7, 2005.

Juul D, Scully JH, Scheiber SC: Achieving board certification in psychiatry: a cohort study. Am J Psychiatry 160:563–565, 2003

Scheiber SC: Balancing validity and reliability by using live patients, in Assessing Clinical Reasoning: The Oral Examination and Alternative Methods. Edited by Mancall EL, Bashook PG. Evanston, IL, American Board of Medical Specialties, 1995

Scheiber SC: Graduate psychiatric education, in Kaplan and Sadock's Comprehensive Textbook of Psychiatry, 8th Edition. Edited by Sadock BJ, Sadock VA. Philadelphia, PA, Lippincott Williams and Wilkins, 2005, pp 3931–3943

Scheiber SC, Kramer TAM, Adamowski S (eds): Core Compentencies for Psychiatric Practice: What Clinicians Need to Know. Washington, DC, American Psychiatric Publishing, 2003

Shore JH, Scheiber SC (eds): Certification, Recertification, and Lifetime Learning in Psychiatry. Washington, DC, American Psychiatric Press, 1994

# Being a Good Mentor and Colleague

Linda L. M. Worley, M.D.

Jonathan F. Borus, M.D.

Donald M. Hilty, M.D.

Relationships with colleagues are an essential part of all academic careers. They foster enjoyable collaboration, learning from and with others, and academic productivity, and they add a social element to one's work. In particular, an effective mentoring relationship is critical in providing advice on how and when to do what in one's academic career. Each institution has its own set of written rules and requirements for promotion and tenure and its own unspoken institutional culture. A good mentor will help you understand both the formal and the informal ways that academia works and will help you stay focused on activities consistent with your career aspirations. In addition, association with a good mentor will enhance your reputation. Mentorship has been long recognized as vital to a mentee's achieving higher levels of career satisfaction, promotion (Majure et al. 1994; Roche 1979; Schapira et al. 1992), publications (Bland and Schmitz 1986), confidence in his or her capabilities (Levenson et al. 1991), research productivity (Steiner et al. 2004), and financial success (Roche 1979).

## DEFINITIONS

A *mentor* is an active partner in an ongoing relationship with a more junior colleague (his or her *mentee*) for the primary purpose of nurturing the mentee's optimal personal and professional development. A mentor serves as a teacher, role model, resource, advisor, supporter, and advocate (Sachdeva 1996). In a positive mentorship pairing, this relationship is mutually beneficial and evolves over time, and the mentee often becomes a valuable colleague to the mentor (Majure et al. 1994).

## TYPES OF MENTORS AND MENTORING RELATIONSHIPS

Mentoring may be divided into two types defined by the functional role the mentor is asked to play. *Developmental mentors* serve as overall guides to a field as well as address the specific personal and professional goals of the mentee. Such mentors are usually in the same field as their mentee and often at the same institution so that the pair can meet on a regular basis and are likely to see one another informally at university or departmental meetings. In addition, professionals often also require *technical mentors,* again usually at the same site, to help the mentee master specific skills (e.g., grant writing, laboratory techniques, specific teaching skills). It is possible, but often not the case, that the same person may perform both of these different mentoring roles. If necessary, both developmental and technical mentors can function from a distance if appropriate mentors (e.g., women, minorities, those with specialized interests) are not available locally.

Mentoring relationships are formed in different ways. Some departments have formal mentoring programs in which senior faculty are officially assigned to more junior faculty or trainees in need of mentoring (Levy et al. 2004). These relationships are time-limited, with specific expectations regarding frequency of meetings and overall goals and expectations. In such programs, mentors may be given a variety of incentives (e.g., monetary reimbursement for expenses for entertaining the mentee, the possibility for mentoring awards, institutional recognition for academic citizenship). Mentoring may also grow out of the vital role it plays in productive research careers. Lab chiefs typically assume a technical mentoring role for the graduate students and postdoctoral students who work in their labs, and the K-awards (National Institutes of Health grants for physician career development) build in funding for such ongoing mentorship (Steiner et al. 2004). Mentoring may also develop naturally between individuals with shared professional interests. During the course of an academic career, it is possible to develop a multitude of mentoring relationships of different types.

Below are two tables that describe the ideal mentor (Table 26–1) and mentee (Table 26–2).

---

**TABLE 26–1.** The ideal mentor

---

*The ideal mentor…*

1. Believes in you.
2. Is psychologically mature.
3. Listens to your dreams and facilitates you reaching them.
4. Gives honest feedback, both good and bad.
5. Promotes your career; pushes you to publish, present your work, and participate in research opportunities.
6. Facilitates your professional networking.
7. Teaches things that books cannot.
8. Celebrates your successes.
9. Is *not* exploitative, smothering, or overly controlling.

---

*Source.* Bhagia and Tinsley 2000; Juul and Scheiber 2004; Levy et al. 2004; Majure et al. 1994; Steiner et al. 2004.

---

**TABLE 26–2.** The ideal mentee

---

*The ideal mentee…*

1. Is courteous, hard-working, and reliable.
2. Takes responsibility for his or her own growth and development.
3. Is efficient and respectful of time.
4. Asks burning questions.
5. Is responsive to advice from mentor.
6. Is enthusiastic and eager to contribute to ongoing work or projects.
7. Expresses gratitude.
8. Is *not* greedy, demanding, clinging, or ungrateful.

---

# PRACTICAL TIPS

## Finding Your Own Mentor

While it may flatter some to be pursued by a potential mentee, successful academicians rarely have a lot of free time. Keep this in mind as you request to meet with a potential mentor. Do your homework ahead of time by reading your mentor's work and understanding his or her breadth of expertise. Send a letter of interest and your CV in advance of telephoning your mentor's assistant to set up a time to talk. Be direct and respectful, explaining that you are interested in their boss's work and that you are eager to find a 30-minute window to meet to talk about the possibility of mentorship. Recognize that the most successful mentoring relationships contain an element of personal chemistry or shared interests. Utilize this first meeting to compare interests and to consider whether a mentoring relationship could be mutually beneficial. Meeting this first time doesn't obligate you or your potential mentor to ever meet again.

## Mentee Etiquette

For a mentee to benefit fully from a mentoring relationship, it is important to abide by unspoken expectations. Appropriate mentee etiquette is as follows:

- Be prepared and arrive early for meetings.
- Dress and talk professionally.
- Turn off your pager (if possible) and cell phone.
- For the initial meeting, bring a polished copy of your CV and a one-page summary of your immediate goals, your current strategy to achieve these goals, and one or two points on how the mentor could be helpful.
- Come prepared with specific questions.
- Be direct, greet warmly, and express gratitude.
- When your mentor extends significant time and effort on your behalf, reciprocate with a thoughtful gesture.
- When invited to participate in some capacity, give your best effort and meet deadlines; speak up early if a deadline is not feasible.
- Return the gift to junior colleagues by becoming a mentor.

## Mentor Etiquette

The role of mentor also is more effective and satisfying if the mentor abides by the following etiquette:

- Be available and responsive to your mentee.
- Be on time.
- Avoid interruptions during meetings.
- Share appropriate resources as indicated.
- Maintain friendly, professional boundaries.
- Be fair about authorship and credit for work done together—generosity to your mentee is an indicator of your professional success.
- Recognize that your mentee's success is a reflection of your mentoring—never compete.
- Open doors for your mentee to opportunities in your department

and appropriate professional organizations.

- Promote your mentee in the direction of his or her career aspirations, which may be different from yours.
- Monitor the academic progress of your mentee and provide helpful feedback.
- Observe confidentiality (i.e., avoid discussion of your mentee with others in the department).

## SMART STRATEGIES

*...for mentors to recommend and mentees to follow:*

- Be certain that mentees fully grasp the general requirements for promotion and tenure early in their academic appointment.
- Require mentees to build and maintain a professional file composed of the necessary components for promotion and tenure (e.g., teaching and supervisory evaluations, reprints, time and effort devoted to committee work, etc.).
- Invite mentees to participate in academic writing and the journal review process, including co-reviewing manuscripts.
- Actively facilitate opportunities for mentees to participate in writing projects with others.

## QUESTIONS TO DISCUSS WITH A MENTOR OR COLLEAGUE

1. How can I achieve my career aspirations and specific goals? What is an appropriate timeline for these goals?
2. What are the necessary tasks to achieve promotion?
3. What are the details of this institution's promotion process? How can I let the department chair know that I am ready to be promoted? What is included in promotion and tenure packet documents, submission deadlines, etc.?
4. In what proportions do I distribute my efforts (clinical, teaching, research)? Are these figures congruent with my career goals? If not, how can I renegotiate a reallocation of effort?
5. How can I achieve balance between my professional and personal life?

## REFERENCES

Bhagia J, Tinsley J: The mentoring partnership. Mayo Clin Proc 75:535–537, 2000
Bland C, Schmitz C: Characteristics of the successful researcher and implications for faculty development. J Med Educ 61:22–31, 1986

Juul D, Scheiber S: Fostering Leadership for the Future: A How-To on Mentoring. Albuquerque, NM, Association for Academic Psychiatry, 2004

Levenson W, Kaufman K, Clark B, et al: Mentors and role models for women in academic medicine. West J Medicine 154(4):423–426, 1991

Levy B, Katz J, Wolf MA, et al: Initiative in mentoring to promote residents' and faculty members' careers. Acad Med 79:845–850, 2004

Majure J, Aylward C, Cranmer S, et al: Pocket Mentor: A Manual for Surgical Interns and Residents. Westmont, IL, Association of Women Surgeons, 1994

Roche G: Much ado about mentors. Harvard Business Review 1:14–28, 1979

Sachdeva A: Preceptorship, mentorship, and the adult learner in medical and health sciences education. J Cancer Educ 11:131–136, 1996

Schapira M, Kalet A, Schwartz MD, et al: Mentorship in general internal medicine: investment in our future. J Gen Intern Med 7:248–251, 1992

Steiner J, Curtis P, Lanphear BP, et al: Assessing the role of influential mentors in the research development of primary care fellows. Acad Med 79:865–872, 2004

## ADDITIONAL RESOURCES

American Association of Medical Colleges Web site. Available at: http://www.aamc.org/members/facultydev/sept04/start.htm. Accessed March 7, 2005.

Association for Academic Psychiatry [AAP Web site]. Available at: http://www.academicpsychiatry.org. Accessed March 7, 2005.

Janet Bickel and Associates: Career development and executive coach. Available at: http://www.janetbickel.com. Accessed March 7, 2005.

UC Davis School of Medicine Mentoring Program Guide: Mentoring program guide for selecting a mentor and establishing a mentoring relationship. Available at: http://med-acaffairs.ucdavis.edu/development/Mentor_Guide.htm. Accessed March 7, 2005.

University of Arkansas for Medical Sciences Faculty Development Speakers [UAMS Web site]. Available at: http://www.uams.edu/cmefa/faculty_affairs/Career_Advice.asp. Accessed March 7, 2005.

# Networking

Laura Weiss Roberts, M.D., M.A.

Donald M. Hilty, M.D.

Deborah J. Hales, M.D.

Supportive relationships with colleagues are a source of great personal fulfillment for many of us and oftentimes can lead to opportunities for professional development and growth. The process of initiating, nurturing, and sustaining these relationships early in one's career is especially important. Referred to as *networking,* pursuing relationships with people outside of our usual context has helped foster careers and facilitate professional advancement throughout history. This chapter discusses some advantages to two kinds of networking, and it provides some guidance for how to approach this process of connecting with others, individually (*primary networking*) or through group activities (*secondary networking*)—even if you are relatively isolated, shy, or worried about coming across as self-promoting.

## PRIMARY NETWORKING

Primary networking involves developing meaningful personal connections with individual people you encounter in your professional life. This is a worthwhile process. It allows a professional person to compare experiences, to find and offer encouragement, to learn more about the responsibilities and activities of others, and to collaborate on efforts of mutual concern. When interacting with colleagues regionally and nationally, one can step out of a local, departmental, or institutional environment to gain perspective on one's strengths and value in relation to one's peer group. For some individuals, networking will stimulate new ideas and serve as an opportunity for brainstorming. For others, it will help to forge a professional identity, for instance, as a clinical subspecialist or as an educator with a particular scholarly focus. Yet others will find it helpful in understanding and gaining access to interdisciplinary expertise or technical support, for instance, when thinking about undertaking a new research project, designing a new course curriculum, or creating a new academic program.

Primary networking may be focused on specific interests in areas of research, education, administration, or clinical care. For example, an educator with interest in psychotherapy training who has developed a training module might seek out others to review it. He or she may also ask others to implement it in order to systematically collect data. This is how oncology first started doing clinical trials on less common cancers—by collating teams from across the country to study outcomes with interventions. Another example would be putting together a conference on medical education: participants would come from key organizations to participate in task forces at a summit, pooling together in groups by interest (e.g., a group based in the members' expertise on how to use innovative technology in various curricula).

## Advantages for Early Career Faculty

Primary networking benefits people in many different roles and disciplines, and its advantages may vary according to one's position in academia. For medical students and residents, networking may introduce the best person to give a letter of recommendation, offer appropriate research opportunities, and act as a role model for a clinical or research career. For residents making the transition to fellowship or faculty roles, primary networking can help to identify good-fit positions. For midcareer and later-career faculty, networking offers the chance to find collaborators and mentees as well as to identify continued opportunities for skills development, leadership, and professional contribution.

Three advantages to primary networking for the early career academic faculty member are worth special attention. First, collegial relationships of this nature give emotional support. Being an academically committed faculty member with substantial clinical, educational, scholarly, and administrative duties and seemingly impossible expectations to

meet in order to be successful is a very hard job. It is difficult for one's immediate colleagues to provide all of the support that is needed because
they, at best, are experiencing similar pressures in the local environment
and, at worst, sometimes feel like competitors, not colleagues. It is also
difficult to gain enough support from supervisors, division directors, or
from the department chair, who may be responsible for some of the pressures to perform that a new faculty member naturally feels. Talking with
a colleague of similar rank, but not from your local setting, is a wonderful
way to give and receive encouragement, advice, and kindness.

Second, the process of seeking and sustaining collegial relationships
has unexpectedly positive consequences over time that are hard to appreciate at the outset. For instance, a person you encounter at a conference may write a letter of support for your promotion a few years from
now; another person may become a trusted advisor or research collaborator. Yet another may offer you an appointment in a professional organization, or give you a hot tip about a new job or a grant opportunity.
Each of the authors of this chapter could share numerous stories of how
a chance meeting with a colleague years ago led to something positive—
this book itself is a great example of this! Similarly, you may offer ideas,
suggestions, and concrete efforts to help your colleagues elsewhere.

The third key reason for the early career faculty member to give time
and attention to networking is finding a mentor (see Chapter 26 in this volume). We believe that one's need for mentoring never really stops because
mentoring requirements evolve and grow as one's interests, commitments,
and skills develop. Very successful academic faculty members will often
identify a stable of outstanding mentors who helped them to be effective
and to grow at different points in their careers. For instance, one of the authors can identify sustained and sincere mentoring relationships with a 9th-
grade biology teacher, a college history professor, a medical school professor (the most robust of the relationships), a supervisor turned friend, a departmental colleague, two colleagues from other institutions, a vice-chair,
three department chairs, an editor, two National Institutes of Health program officers, four fellow officers in professional organizations, and (at
least) three deans.

## SECONDARY NETWORKING

*Secondary networking* pertains to working with colleagues in groups. There
are many things we are asked to do for our workplaces, departments, state
organizations (e.g., nonprofit granting agencies), and national organizations to which we may belong. Sometimes we enjoy and find value in these

activities, and other times, frankly, these assignments simply represent more work in an already fragile, burdened schedule. However, these activities present opportunities for collaboration and can transition into venues for primary networking—for these reasons alone they are of great value in our professional development.

Consider, for example, an invitation to review proposals for a nonprofit organization in another state, or a request to review articles for a journal. These may seem like chores in that they require a lot of time and energy spent in an activity with no immediate benefit. (And, after all, how many nights can you go without sleep?!) However, it is a real privilege to be able to see proposals and manuscripts at various stages of development and of various quality; this is an outstanding learning experience, the lessons of which can be easily applied to your own work. Moreover, if you work closely with the agency or the journal, they may value your "good citizenship" and keep you in mind for future opportunities (e.g., serving as a paid consultant or being appointed to an editorial board) or pass along your name to others, where your efforts may also lead to benefits of immediate value to you.

## WHAT TO DO, AND NOT DO, IN NETWORKING

The activities involved in networking (see Table 27–1) may be very easy and natural for some people. These are the people who like going to conferences, enjoy chatting with others, seek out novel professional situations, are willing to take on responsibility or risk (e.g., of serving on a high-visibility committee), and want to keep in touch with colleagues just because it is fun or interesting. For others, this set of activities sounds like yet another form of protracted misery.

For natural networkers, the challenge will be to manage overcommitment and to be sure to deliver on promises made in networking encounters. For those who find networking much harder, the challenge will be to stretch oneself a bit and to find the right venues for connecting with others in a way that feels genuine, tolerable, fruitful, or possibly even halfway comfortable. This is particularly true for the early career faculty member who has been in only one or two institutional settings and has made few professional acquaintances outside of his or her department. Whether it comes easily or not, undertaking and fostering collegial relationships through primary and secondary networking requires effort and attention in order to be effective.

There are a couple of things to keep in mind that are particularly helpful in facilitating collegial relationships. First, put yourself in situa-

---

**TABLE 27-1.** Opportunities for networking

---

1. Organizations: Get involved (e.g., APA, ABPN, AAP, AADPRT, ADMSEP, APM).
2. Writing: Collaborate with others on articles, case reports, reviews, and books.
3. Educational projects: Compare notes and share resources with others (e.g., curricula and teaching methods).
4. Programming: Join in (e.g., work on program committees, editorial boards).
5. Presenting: Share your data, experiences, practices, and programs (e.g., through posters, panels, talks, and committees).
6. Nominating: Help your colleagues attain institutional, regional, and national awards.
7. Communicating: Even if you cannot stand small talk!

---

*Note.* AADPRT=American Association of Directors of Psychiatry Residency Training; ABPN=American Board of Psychiatry and Neurology; ADMSEP= Association of Directors of Medical Student Education in Psychiatry; APA=American Psychiatric Association APM=Academy of Psychosomatic Medicine.

tions where you are more likely to have meaningful interactions with colleagues that you find interesting. For instance, if you love teaching, you may wish to attend conferences and become involved with organizations that have an educational focus, such as the American Association of Directors of Psychiatry Residency Training (AADPRT), the Association for Academic Psychiatry (AAP), the Association of Directors of Medical Student Education in Psychiatry (ADMSEP), the Academy of Psychosomatic Medicine (APM), and others. While gaining content expertise in the area of teaching, you may also find like-minded colleagues from various institutions across the country and will more readily find things to discuss. It will be natural to exchange e-mail addresses and phone numbers, to share ideas, to compare curricula, to recommend resources, and later to check in with one another on common interests. An interaction that may start as awkward and superficial small talk at an overcrowded reception thus becomes a spontaneous, authentic, and substantive collegial relationship over time.

Second, be friendly (even if you are shy) and, to the extent that you can possibly manage it, be generous to the colleagues you meet. Put your focus on being supportive and on truly giving to your colleagues. Invite colleagues to help you put together poster and panel presentations. Be the co-author who always delivers. Remember to nominate your colleagues for awards and honors, and always remember to thank those who have helped you. These things do much to build a reservoir of good will. On the other hand, all of us have been on the short end of an interaction with a fellow professional whose only objective, it seemed, was to make us feel inadequate. Similarly, all of us have had interactions where we felt someone wanted something from us, rather than bringing some reciprocal or mutual good to an interaction. Watching your own motivations, and seeking out professional interactions where you can serve to help your colleague as well as possibly find some personal benefit, are both very important to effective networking and, more importantly, to building valuable and sustenance-providing collegial relationships across your professional lifetime.

There are a couple of things to avoid when networking. First, it is vital to not criticize in an adamant manner your program, your director, your department chair, or your colleagues. Networking is not the same as venting; while it may feel like a relief to let off some steam about your immediate work environment, networking has no confidentiality boundaries—or practically so—and occurs in a relatively small academic community. What you say will often be shared with others; indeed, in one way, this is an important function of networking. It is vital to engage in networking in a manner that seeks to improve your reputation and to connect positively with others—not garner a reputation as a curmudgeon, a poor team player, or, worse yet, an unprofessional colleague.

In addition, it is important to not neglect what might best be described as subtle issues related to power in networking. Academic organizations, professional societies, and clinical and research institutions are typically hierarchical, and networking activities sometimes highlight where one fits in the scheme of things—including the prejudices that may come along with these perceptions. With discussions of being an instructor versus assistant professor, a clinician-educator versus tenure track faculty member, a generalist versus a subspecialist, at a public versus private institution, in a more modest department versus a more robust department, and the like, come many opportunities to become competitive or defensive. This does much to undo the potential good of networking. Discussions of this sort, on the other hand, can be used as positive opportunities to educate colleagues about the true strengths and disadvantages of your particular situation and to learn about those of others.

Another power-related issue in networking is the importance of connecting with people in different roles, ranks, and disciplines. Networking with administrative support staff, as well as with doctoral-level professionals, is vital. If you only network with people in high-ranking positions and are inattentive or dismissive toward peers or people seen as lower in the professional hierarchy, this pattern gets noticed very quickly and will not serve you well.

Finally, individuals who are in empowered positions (e.g., officers in professional organizations, faculty of higher academic rank, mentors, editors, and accomplished educators and scholars) may not always understand the impact of their words or nonverbal expressions on colleagues who look up to them. Just as signs of encouragement and affirmation can take on extraordinary importance, negative or unthinking remarks can, unfortunately, take on disproportionate weight. Attending to these aspects of networking will help ensure that interactions remain on good footing and have a positive impact.

In sum, collegial interactions may offer great support, sustenance, and rewards. They require generosity, attention, and effort, and are of particular importance in the professional development of the early career faculty member. Encouraging others and receiving encouragement, giving and getting support, opening doors to others, and having doors opened to you are companion activities that may start with networking but result in deep, prolonged, and valued relationships.

## SMART STRATEGIES

- Be friendly, reach out, stay in touch, be generous, and say "thanks."
- Make yourself available when work needs to be done or when colleagues need support.
- Be quick to give your contact information to colleagues.
- If you are a natural networker, balance your commitments and be sure to deliver on your promises.
- If you are not a natural networker, stretch yourself a bit and find optimal opportunities for genuine interaction with colleagues.
- Pay attention to power issues in your interactions with colleagues.
- See networking as an opportunity to build positive collegial relationships and a positive reputation among your colleagues.

## QUESTIONS TO DISCUSS WITH A MENTOR OR COLLEAGUE

1. Which professional societies and organizations are a good fit for networking with interested and interesting colleagues?
2. Who in my immediate environment might I reach out to, and why?
3. Can you give me some examples of how networking with colleagues has led to positive developments? Any examples of negative outcomes related to networking?

## ADDITIONAL RESOURCES

Gladwell M: The Tipping Point: How Little Things Can Make a Big Difference. Boston, MA, Little, Brown, 2000

Heim P, Golant SK: Hardball for Women: Winning at the Game of Business. New York, Plume, 1993

Kouzes JM, Posner BZ: The Leadership Challenge, 3rd Edition. San Francisco, CA, Jossey-Bass, 2002

# CHAPTER 28

# Taking Care of Yourself

Blythe A. Corbett, Ph.D.

The academic career path is an exciting, demanding endeavor, which at times can lead to stress. For the purpose of this chapter, *stress* is defined as a psychological, emotional, and biological tension resulting from a perceived threat to the normal processes or integrated functions of an organism. A threat exists when the perceived environment is in contrast to the expectations of the individual. The subsequent stress response is an active process, which can be both adaptive and harmful, that seeks to respond to the threat or changes in the environment while allowing for optimum bodily function or homeostasis (Cannon 1929). *Homeostasis* refers to the stability of physiological systems that are maintained within an optimal range to sustain life. Hans Selye (1956), the father of stress research, recognized that the response to stress is adaptive because it seeks to preserve life; yet it can be harmful through severe or prolonged exposure to challenge.

The demands on a young academic psychiatrist, although usually not life-threatening, can be relentless. *Allostasis,* which supports homeostasis, is the process of achieving stability through change (McEwen and Wingfield 2003). This suggests that when a demand has not been removed or neutralized, maintaining homeostasis may be a persistent

I would like to thank Laura Weiss Roberts, M.D., for her support and guidance on this chapter; Patricio Ayala, M.D., for his assistance in gathering and organizing various manuscripts for review; and Brian Jacobson for his contribution of the graphic models.

source of wear on the system (Sterling and Eyer 1988). Thus, the endurance of stress, or *allostatic load*, considers the cost of persistent, psychosocial stressors that may contribute to long-term damage to health and psychological well-being (McEwen and Stellar 1993). In other words, these psychosocial stressors compete for coping resources and reduce the ability of the person to cope with new demands (Lovallo 2005).

However, despite the acknowledged stressors and consequences impinging on health care professionals, topics of self-care and physician impairment are typically not included in professional training or practice (Miller and McGowen 2000). *Physician impairment* refers to the presence of a mental, physical, or substance-related disorder in the practitioner that interferes with his or her ability to practice medicine both safely and competently (Council of Ethical and Judicial Affairs 2002). The precise prevalence of such impairment among physicians is difficult to determine because of self-medication, a failure to seek health care, concern of stigmatization, fear of losing medical licensure, and other personal factors. Substance abuse prevalence among physicians is likely comparable to that in the general population (Brewster 1986), but it may be more problematic because of the consequential risk to public safety and the inherent resistance among physicians to seeking help (Weir 2000). In regard to other issues such as suicide, physicians do show increased vulnerability. A recent meta-analysis of suicide rates among physicians showed modest to high elevations in suicide rates for men and for women as compared to the general population (Schernhammer and Colditz 2004).

In an attempt to better understand the origins of physician impairment, several investigators have examined the health issues of medical students. In a large-scale study of physical and mental health concerns among 1,027 students at nine U.S. medical schools, it was found that 90% reported a variety of health concerns and 47% reported at least one mental health- or substance-related issue (Roberts et al. 2001). The prevalence rate of alcoholism and substance abuse among medical students has been reported to range from 7% to 18% (Baldwin et al. 1991; Flaherty and Richman 1993; Schwartz et al. 1990). However, despite high rates of health concerns and mental health issues, many students fail to obtain necessary care and instead choose maladaptive coping strategies (Roberts et al. 2001).

The transition from medical school and residency to academia is replete with rewards and the sense of accomplishment. Nevertheless, the academic environment is filled with potential sources of stress from deadlines and competing demands that involve both immediate and future consequences (see Figure 28–1). Occupations associated with a high level of demand and a low level of control are associated with increased stress and consequently tend to lead to more stress-related illnesses (Smith et al. 1978). In a multivariate analysis of general practitioners, four primary stressors were identified as predictive of job dissatisfaction and a lack of mental well-being: interference with family life, persistent interruptions at work and home, practice administration, and job and patient expectations (Cooper et al. 1989). In another investigation, similar factors were identified, in addition to specific concerns related to competence among doctors early in practice (Simpson and Grant 1991). Although there are different types of stress, within this context we focus on two primary types of psychological stress that pertain to factors of control and expectation.

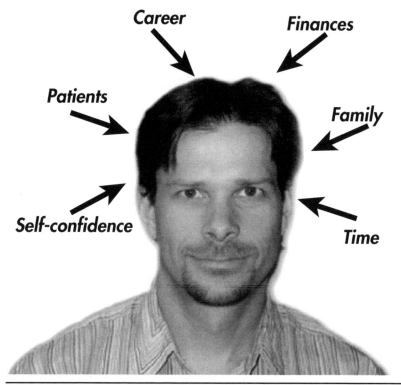

**FIGURE 28–1.** Competing concerns and responsibilities in an early career faculty member.

## CONTROL

The absence of control or the loss of real or perceived control can elicit either a search for immediate affirmation of control or an effortful attempt to exert control over the situation. One's ability to cope is influenced by the ability to exert some control over a situation. It has been postulated that individuals who have a more internal locus of control and believe that they have power over their lives may be better able to cope with stress than those who believe that fate, luck, or the actions of others determine their circumstances (Rotter 1966).

Research with older individuals has shown that control over even minor matters may have major positive consequences (Rodin and Langer 1977). Conversely, extreme frustration can lead to learned helplessness in which an organism learns to do nothing even when it would be possible to exert control over a stressful situation (Seligman 1977). A case in point is physician burnout, which consists of mental, emotional, and physical exhaustion resulting from long-term involvement in situations that are emotionally demanding. It is not simply the stress that leads to physician burnout. Rather, burnout results when stress continuously outweighs the sense of effectiveness and reward (Hirsch 1999). The conditions of the workplace are primary determinants of a physician's physical and mental well-being (Williams et al. 2002). Thus, these investigations suggest that one must maintain a certain level of control in the workplace, which may mean being involved in choices, decisions, and endeavors that have implications for one's career.

## NOVELTY AND VIOLATION OF EXPECTATIONS

Another significant source of stress is the violation of expectations that an individual has in a given circumstance, or the *novelty of a situation*. Embarking on a new career in academia entails certain expectations, the reality of which may or may not match your prior idea of academic life. Psychological stress may result from the dissonance between what was anticipated and the demands of the new experience. The stress system, and in particular the hypothalamic-pituitary-adrenal (HPA) axis, responds consistently to new or unfamiliar events (Hennessey and Levine 1979). The violation of expectations activates a cascade of neural and endocrine responses that result in the release of adrenal hormones. During times of stress, the autonomic (sympathetic, parasympathetic, and enteric nervous system) and endocrine (adrenocortical response) systems are activated. The major stress hormones include epinephrine, which reinforces the actions of the sympathetic nerves, and cortisol, which plays a role during normal metabolic activity and is elevated during periods of stress. The biological outcome of the stress response for the individual is determined by the individual's ability to react, resist, and adapt to the source of stress (Selye 1956). To speak in the vernacular, your ability to manage the day-to-day stressors relies on your capacity to cope with ever-increasing and changing demands. Mental health providers must be aware of and responsive to their own needs and limitations and must plan their personal and professional lives accordingly (Whitfield 1980).

## COPING AND RESOURCES

It is anticipated that this book will assist you in managing the new changes and challenges of beginning an academic career. Nevertheless, we recognize that the novelty may make you feel threatened or vulnerable. Specifically, "threat exists when one perceives that his or her self-esteem is in jeopardy; vulnerability exists when the lack of resources creates a potentially threatening or harmful situation" (Brannon and Feist 1992, p. 60); that is, vulnerability presents the potential for perceiving a threat. Therefore, your ability to cope may be determined, in part, by your available resources. Resources may be physical or social, but their influence and importance is determined by the psychological and emotional salience tied to them.

Coping is an effortful process. It requires persistent effort to manage the perceived stressors. The ability to cope depends on numerous resources: health and energy, positive belief, problem-solving skills, social skills, social support, and material resources (Lazarus and Folkman 1984) (see Figure 28–2).

### Health and Energy

It is a common belief, supported by extensive research, that healthy and robust individuals are better able to cope with both internally and externally imposed demands. Therefore, maintaining a healthy lifestyle of regular exercise can allow you not only to expend more energy and stay in shape but also to inoculate your body through repeated exposure to moderate levels of physical stress. Thus, exercise provides an illustration of the idea that exposure to a stressor can increase the organism's ability to adapt and cope with the stressor in the future through adaptation (Selye 1956).

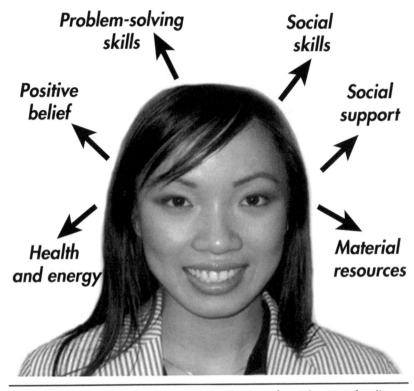

**FIGURE 28–2.**    Strengths for responding to stress for early career faculty members.

Another important factor in health is sleep, which many learn in medical school to be a luxury rather than a necessity. Despite its taxing effects, sleep deprivation is typically considered a consequence rather than a cause of stress. The effects of a lack of sleep are typically more psychological than physical and generally do not pose a health hazard. Nevertheless, sleep deprivation may reduce motivation (Webb and Cartwright 1978) as well as lead to inattention and difficulty concentrating, which can increase the risk of accidents (Akerstedt 1988). Maintaining good sleep hygiene that results in being well rested may contribute to an increased feeling of wellness and productivity.

## Self-Efficacy

Your belief, or lack thereof, in your own ability to perform is a critical factor in determining your response to stress. *Self-efficacy* refers to the confidence that one has in one's ability to perform behaviors that are necessary to produce the desired outcomes in a particular situation (Bandura 1977, 1986). Adopting a mental set consistent with self-efficacy, in which one is able to acquire and maintain the skills necessary to perform a given task results in more positive consequences.

## Problem-Solving Skills

The life of a psychiatrist or health care provider by definition involves conflicts that require excellent problem-solving skills for their resolution. Thus, the ability to create solutions to simple and complex problems through the utilization of both internal and external resources can help determine success (also see Chapter 8 in this volume).

## Social Skills

*Social skills* refers to a broad repertoire of behaviors that allow one to interact with others in a meaningful and respectful manner. Among the many individual skills associated with socialization are the ability to perceive the actions of others, relate to them, and respond in an appropriate way. In academia, as in other complex social systems, the impact of a stressor depends heavily on the way in which the individual perceives the situation as it involves other people, manages his or her accompanying emotions, and selects an adaptive response.

## Social Support

The concept of social support involves the feeling of being accepted and supported by family, friends, and others. To some extent, social support can provide a buffer that protects against the negative consequences of stress (Cassel 1976; Kaplan 1977). As mental health professionals, we know the importance of social support in the amelioration of mental and physical illness. Similarly, the presence of social support can assist us in better meeting the demands of our career. Social support includes four primary factors: 1) emotional concern (expressing empathy and caring); 2) instrumental aid (giving and receiving assistance); 3) information (giving and receiving advice, directions, and suggestions); and 4) appraisal (feedback from the other person's appraisal) (House 1984). It is of great importance that we "take some of our own medicine" from time to time and seek the essential support that our social networks can provide.

It is also important to highlight that our career development paths, professional choices and related rewards, stressors, and consequences do not occur in isolation. We must be aware of the impact that we have on those around us. In particular, we must acknowledge and remember that the social support we seek must also be nurtured and reciprocated among our partnerships, family, and close relationships.

## Materials

In addition to the psychological and social factors mentioned, many physical and practical factors can reduce stress, contribute to a healthier existence, and allow one to reach full potential. Maslow (1943; 1970) proposed a hierarchy of needs, in which physiological, security, social, and esteem needs must be met in order for one to become a fulfilled or actualized human being. In his model, the material needs are fundamental and may determine one's ability to achieve sufficiency. Thus, we must care for our basic needs first and learn to become practical and inventive by making use of available tools and resources to achieve success. The fundamental purpose of this guide as a tool is to provide you with many ideas that can aid in the establishment, maintenance, and advancement of your career.

Lastly, there are periods in all of our lives when the stress and demands of our life may become too great and require that we seek professional help. It is the hope that the profession has instilled in you the identification and need for psychiatric treatment when warranted. Therefore, it is respectfully recommended that you be your own best support and refer yourself for help if the need arises.

## CONCLUSIONS

Many demands impinge on the young academic that may contribute to high levels of stress. It is imperative to keep a certain level of control in the workplace, which includes being involved in choices, decisions, and endeavors that have implications for your career. As mental health professionals, we must be aware of and responsive to our own needs lest we become unable to provide the necessary care for others, and we must plan our personal and professional lives accordingly. It is helpful to remember that coping is an effortful and persistent process. It is suggested that a variety of internal resources (e.g., positive belief) and external resources (e.g., social support) can assist you in managing and facilitating your academic career.

## SMART STRATEGIES

- Accurately identify sources of stress in your professional life.
- Identify your strengths and vulnerabilities in handling stress.
- Engage in active self-care (e.g., good sleep and nutrition).
- Adopt a mental set of positive self-beliefs.
- Cultivate your adaptive skills.

## QUESTIONS TO DISCUSS WITH A MENTOR OR COLLEAGUE

1. Does the department have a career management program that provides guidance, responsiveness, and support for young faculty?
2. What do you consider to be the key stressors in beginning an academic career?
3. What are some of the coping strategies that you use or endorse to help manage the stress of an academic career?
4. Are there formalized resources and opportunities established for young faculty to meet each other for mutual support?
5. What are the vacation and sick leave policies in the department for young faculty?
6. Do you know a good gym, massage therapist, or walking path?

## REFERENCES

Akerstedt T: Sleepiness as a consequence of shiftwork. Sleep 11:17–34, 1988

Baldwin DC Jr, Hughes PH, Conard SE, et al: Substance use among senior medical students: a survey of 23 medical schools. JAMA 265:2074–2078, 1991

Bandura A: Social Learning Theory. Englewood Cliffs, NJ, Prentice-Hall, 1977

Bandura A: Social Foundations of Thought and Action: A Social Cognitive Theory. Englewood Cliffs, NJ, Prentice-Hall, 1986

Brannon L, Feist J: Health Psychology: An Introduction to Behavior and Health. Belmont, CA, Wadsworth, 1992

Brewster J: Prevalence of alcohol and other drug problems among physicians. JAMA 255:1913–1920, 1986

Cannon WB: Bodily Changes in Pain, Hunger, Fear and Rage, 2nd Edition. New York, Appleton, 1929

Cassel J: The contribution of the social environment to host resistance. Am J Epidemiol 104:107–123, 1976

Cooper CL, Rout U, Faragher B: Mental health, job satisfaction, and job stress among general practitioners. BMJ 11:366–370, 1989

Council of Ethical and Judicial Affairs: Code of Medical Ethics. Chicago, IL, American Medical Association, 2002

Flaherty JA, Richman JA: Substance use and addiction among medical students, residents, and physicians. Psychiatr Clin North Am 16:189–197, 1993

Hennessey JW, Levine S: Stress, arousal, and the pituitary-adrenal system: a psychoendocrine hypothesis. Prog Psychobiol Physiol Psychol 8:133–178, 1979

Hirsch G: Physician career management: organizational strategies for the century. Physician Exec 25:30–35, 1999

House JS: Barriers to work stress, I: social support, in Behavioral Medicine: Work, Stress, and Health. Edited by Gentry WD, Benson H, deWolff C. NATO ASI Series D: Behavioural and Social Sciences, No. 19. Dordrecht, The Netherlands, Nijhoff, 1985, pp 157–180

Kaplan GA, Cassel JC, Gore S: Social supports and health. Medical Care 15:47–58, 1977

Lazarus RS, Folkman S: Stress, Appraisal, and Coping. New York, Springer, 1984

Lovallo WR: Stress and Health. Thousand Oaks, CA, Sage, 2005

Maslow AH: A theory of human motivation. Psychol Rev 50:370–396, 1943

Maslow AH: Motivation and personality. New York, Harper, 1970

McEwen BS, Stellar E: Stress and the individual: mechanisms leading to disease. Arch Intern Med 153:2093–2101, 1993

McEwen BS, Wingfield JC: The concept of allostasis in biology and medicine. Horm Behav 43:2–15, 2003

Miller NM, McGowen RK: The painful truth: physicians are not invincible. South Med J 93:966–973, 2000

Roberts LW, Warner TD, Lyketsos C, et al: Perceptions of academic vulnerability associated with personal illness: a study of 1027 students at nine medical schools. Compr Psychiatry 42:1–15, 2001

Rodin J, Langer EJ: Long-term effects of a control-relevant intervention with the institutionalized aged. J Pers Soc Psychol 35: 897–902, 1977

Rotter JB: Generalized expectancies for internal versus external control of reinforcement. Psychol Monogr 80:1–28, 1966

Schernhammer ES, Colditz GA: Suicide rates among physicians: a quantitative and gender assessment (meta-analysis). Am J Psychiatry 161:2295–2302, 2004

Schwartz RH, Lewis DC, Hoffmann NG, et al: Cocaine and marijuana use by medical students before and during medical school. Arch Intern Med 150:883–886, 1990

Seligman BS: Untangling Tarasoff: Tarasoff v. Regents of the University of California. Hastings Law J 29:179–210, 1977

Selye H: The Stress of Life. New York, McGraw-Hill, 1956

Simpson LA, Grant L: Sources and magnitude of job stress among physicians. J Behav Med 14:27–42, 1991

Smith M, Colligan M, Horning RW, et al: Occupational Comparison of Stress-Related Disease Incidence. Cincinnati, OH, National Institute for Occupational Safety and Health, 1978

Sterling P, Eyer J: Allostasis: A New Paradigm to Explain Arousal Pathology, in Handbook of Life Stress, Cognition, and Health. Edited by Fisher S, Reason J. New York, John Wiley, 1988, pp 629–649

Webb WB, Cartwright RD: Sleep and dreams, Pt. 1. Annu Rev Psychol 29:223–252, 1978

Weir E: Substance abuse among physicians. Can Med Assoc J 162:1730, 2000

Whitfield MD: Emotional stresses on the psychotherapist. Can J Psychiatry 25:292–296, 1980

Williams ES, Konrad RR, Linzer M, et al: Physician, practice, and patient characteristics related to primary care physician physical and mental health: results from the Physician Worklife Study. Health Ser Res 27:121–143, 2002

# CHAPTER 29

# Creating a Positive Early Career Environment

Joel Yager, M.D.

Donald M. Hilty, M.D.

There's no such thing as the perfect work environment. All early career psychiatrists encounter work situations that require tweaking, if not major modifications. In this chapter we offer guidance, Internet resources, and readings regarding what early career psychiatrists can do to improve any work situation. These suggestions are meant to go hand in hand with the efforts of faculty members, departments, hospitals, and schools of medicine. Key elements of a positive career environment include 1) defining your general professional direction; 2) increasing competency in psychiatric technical skills; 3) developing general management and administrative skills; 4) establishing a professional community; and 5) taking care of yourself, including managing your time wisely, optimizing mood and affect, and balancing your career with your personal life.

## DEFINING GENERAL PROFESSIONAL DIRECTIONS

Early career activities are tucked into long-term goals. The early career psychiatrist is well served by having a good sense of personal values and passions as well as reasonably well-defined ideas about desired short- and long-term outcomes. A useful activity to help you in defining your professional direction is to actually write out specific objectives to be accomplished in the next year, 2 years, and 5 years regarding work setting, salary and benefits, work hours, productivity, advancement, and integration of career goals with family goals; some suggest drafting a detailed personal mission statement in order to achieve a proper perspective. One useful exercise is to envision several different possible life outcomes at your 90th birthday, taking into account career, family, and community goals, and then work backwards, imagining exactly what intermediary steps would be required to achieve the most desired outcomes. Another is to list (and regularly revise) the 25 things you really want to accomplish during this lifetime. Such iterative long-term goal setting facilitates gaining a better focus on early career and short-term planning.

Within this long-range framework you can focus down on your early career, first by doing a frank self-assessment (with the help of others) of what you know and don't know professionally. This will facilitate creating a further list of psychiatric technical training and general administrative skills needed to foster the desired early successes you have already identified. What specific psychiatric and general administrative proficiencies are essential for professional survival? Which are necessary but not absolutely essential, and which are desirable but optional? What means are available for acquiring those proficiencies, what concrete steps must occur to assure their acquisition, and what sorts of markers or "deliverables" might indicate actual progress toward these goals? To cultivate balance, the list should include personal goals as well as career goals. Table 29–1 provides a whimsical example of an early career goal-setting list.

## INCREASING TECHNICAL PSYCHIATRIC PROFICIENCIES

Each individual needs to assess exactly what specific competencies will be required for early career success, what was not taught (or learned) in residency, and how best to acquire those missing proficiencies. Because concerns about being incompetent are virtually ubiquitous in all but the most narcissistically well-defended young career psychiatrists, there is always more to learn and there are always skills in need of polishing. Deficits may exist in specific psychiatric technical skills that are needed to assume specific roles (e.g., certain types of clinical assessment, psychotherapy or pharmacotherapy training, electroconvulsive therapy training, forensic skills, and research skills), or more general abilities, such as practice management and administrative skills. Modes of skill acquisition range from informal, on-the-job training through good supervision to more formal continuing education programs. Good lifelong learning habits are essential; reading is always worthwhile, particularly in preparation for board examinations, and teaching is always an excellent way to foster learning.

**TABLE 29–1.** One psychiatrist's early career goal setting

| Goal | Essential or optional? | What I will do this year? | Markers of success |
|---|---|---|---|
| **Technical skills** | | | |
| Learn electroconvulsive therapy | Optional | Find someone with whom to apprentice. | Getting privileged |
| Improve psychotherapy skills | Essential | Contact Dr. A for regular private supervision; join a peer-supervision group. | More self-confidence<br>More scheduled hours |
| Improve psychopharmacology skills | Essential | Read journals regularly.<br>Take a continuing medical education course.<br>Attend grand rounds. | More self-confidence<br>More nuanced prescribing |
| **General administrative** | | | |
| Learn to run an office | Essential | Set up regular meetings with Dr. B.<br>Look into online M.B.A. program.<br>Look into weekend courses. | Able to discuss coding, billing, and collections intelligently with business manager and accountant |
| Learn to hire and fire | Essential | Ask Dr. B.<br>Read M.B.A. stuff. | Satisfaction with personnel |
| Make some money | Essential | Attend to basic practice management issues, such as billing and collecting. | Higher bank balance<br>Lower debts |

(continued)

**TABLE 29–1.**    One psychiatrist's early career goal setting *(continued)*

| Goal | Essential or optional? | What I will do this year? | Markers of success |
|---|---|---|---|
| **Professional community** | | | |
| Establish connections for referrals | Optional | Meet regularly and socialize with Drs. C, D. Actively participate in local psychiatric society, hospital staff. | Regular, steady referrals |
| Establish a teaching role | Essential | Join volunteer faculty of medical school or college. | Schedule teaching time in calendar |
| Establish career trajectory | Essential | Identify likely mentors; establish regular get-togethers. Explore early career psychiatrist resources online, at annual regional and national American Psychiatric Association meetings. | Set meetings, goals in calendar |
| **Personal life** | | | |
| Start exercise program | Optional | Join a gym; buy home equipment; build a regular exercise schedule. | Review calendar Look in mirror |
| Have a child | Optional | First meet a partner. | Reflective review Review calendar |
| Learn to paint | Optional | Get a catalogue; join a class; buy some tools; make some time. | Review calendar Art around? |
| Grow up | Essential | Start personal therapy; get a guru. | Inner peace |

## DEVELOPING MANAGEMENT AND ADMINISTRATIVE SKILLS

Although residencies are now paying greater attention to "transition to practice" courses, what is learned in residency generally does not adequately cover all the specifics likely to be encountered either in solo private practice or institutional settings. Consequently, increasing numbers of early career psychiatrists are enrolling in formal courses, workshops, and even M.B.A. or Executive M.B.A. career programs in order to develop the skills necessary for administrative roles in which they find themselves immersed. These skills include decision making, budgeting, accounting and planning, and organizational dynamics such as people management. Current resources on practice management and general administrative skills are listed at the end of this chapter.

## FINDING MENTORS, COLLEAGUES, AND TEAMMATES

Finding and using mentors, colleagues, and teammates is necessary for the early career psychiatrist. A primary duty is to consider a list of the types of mentors and supervisors you will need in fulfilling the career goals you have outlined, regardless of the setting. Mentors may be selected to help you to acquire certain technical skills (e.g., by establishing an apprenticing relationship) or to provide general perspective and guidance (e.g., by knowing the necessary next step in a given endeavor and being able to identify pitfalls and ways of dealing with them, and by giving overall emotional support). For more details on this, see Chapter 26 in this volume, on mentoring, and keep in mind the following: Take the initiative to establish contact; make clear, reasonable requests; respect the mentors' time and resources; and reciprocate appropriately with respect, thanks, or gifts.

Clinical work may be isolating; establishing a network of colleagues for review of cases, consultations, and cross-referrals is necessary in institutional settings as well as in solo practice. Colleagues should be recruited from one's own profession and subspecialty area, others in mental health, and still others that are general health professionals. Local, regional, and national contacts and connections are all helpful, and all may prove useful regarding specific aspects of practicing psychiatry and career building. Locally, regularly scheduled meetings that are held for supervision, continuing education, and social networking help to reduce isolation, increase a sense of community, and provide emotional support (i.e., opportunities for venting), as well as assistance in solving myriad practical problems.

Working as a psychiatrist inevitably requires many skills. The private practitioner increasingly relies on an effective office staff, which may include nurses, therapists, and business managers. To make certain that successful careers are launched, even the solo psychiatric practitioner and consultant will require at least a good accountant and attorney, and probably an estate planner, insurance agent, and banker. In institutional settings, arrays of administrative personnel—secretaries, clerks, and others—are ubiquitous, and skills in personnel appraisal, assessment, and management are required to hire, fire, or contend with staff. Group and organizational dynamics courses, unfortunately not often taught in psychiatric residency programs, offer insights into some of the adverse interpersonal dynamics one is likely to encounter in work settings and a deeper understanding of their meaning. From a practical perspective, the literature on dealing with difficult people and undertaking difficult conversations, listed at the end of this chapter, is well worth reading.

## SELF-MANAGEMENT

*Self-management* involves knowing how to manage your time, your mood, and your affect, as well as knowing how to balance your career and personal life (see Chapters 8 and 28). Studies have shown that physicians who consciously organize their work week and workdays have greater work satisfaction than those who do not (Linn et al. 1985, 1986). General principles of time management include scheduling specific hours (not including for protected time) for returning phone calls or e-mails; for catching up with mail, correspondence, filing, and general administrative activities; and for reading medical journals.

Aside from biology, managing one's mood is largely a function of choosing the right perspective, and choosing proper reference groups. How we think we're doing usually comes down to framing our behavior as compared with something or someone else. The act of creative "perspectivizing" is important for the emotional self-regulation that you necessarily undertake to stay upbeat with respect to your career. During times of distress, it's always good to take a few steps back to realize that your educational and career opportunities have likely ensured that you're among the very fortunate. Such perspective may help uplift you during moments of demoralization and reduce whiny self-pity.

Immediate threats to one's affective calm emanate from several sources at work: unanticipated difficult situations concerning interpersonal conflicts; seemingly impossibly conflicting choices, demands, and situations in which complex decision making is required to determine not only the best alternative but the least worse alternatives; and returning from vacation and facing a mountain of waiting work. Several cognitive self-management strategies may be particularly helpful:

- Albert Ellis's list of irrational assumptions and rational-emotive alternatives (Ellis and Harper 1975) are highly recommended—for example, pushing thoughts to absurd extremes, as in "What's the worst than can happen?" analyses.
- A wise psychiatric administrator once described his management philosophy as having a few guiding principles to provide "vision," but primarily, on a day-to-day basis, "muddling through" (Greenblatt 1978).
- Reentry after a relaxing time away is often experienced as a rude assault of tasks and emotions. Scheduling extra time or deliberately putting one's emotions on hold for 3–5 days after returning may reduce or forestall dysphoria.
- Attention to small things and healthy pleasures in the workplace may go far in keeping one's day-to-day emotions in a healthy state. Are there small changes to make the work environment more pleasant (e.g., furnishing your office with a coffee pot, small refrigerator, better lighting, more comfortable furniture, plants, adornments, music, or better feng shui)? As an early career psychiatrist, make certain to take adequate nutrition, hydration, physical activity, and bathroom breaks during the day.

Attending to family, community, and personal needs in addition to career demands is always a difficult balancing act, particularly for women. Assessing your desires, obligations, resources, and options requires negotiating with your family, your colleagues, and yourself, and iteratively trying things out. Knowing yourself well enough is critical. Although harried early careers may impose numerous conflicting obligations, building in adequate time for personal exercise, needed intimacies, and reflective solitude for creative self-expression or just plain needed down time are valuable investments in your short-term and long-term well-being and success. Useful sources on the general topic of self-management are listed at the end of the chapter.

## SMART STRATEGIES

- Be honest with yourself and appraise your decisions regarding what really matters to you emotionally as well as intellectually; sleep on your decisions, and listen to your gut instincts.

- Make your early career decisions in the context of your current personal life and family needs as well as in the context of your long-term personal and career goals. Don't sacrifice your personal life or family any more than is absolutely necessary to accomplish your professional goals.
- Clarify your major professional gaps and determine how you might most efficiently and effectively master those competencies you will require most immediately.
- Speak directly with anyone who can help answer questions about professional settings, jobs, and situations. In working up your potential early career environments, don't be shy—get on the phone to current and past incumbents as well as anyone else likely to have useful information.

## QUESTIONS TO DISCUSS WITH A MENTOR OR COLLEAGUE

1. As you look back on your early career, what sorts of things do you wish you had done then that you didn't do (i.e., what errors of omission did you make)?
2. As you look back on your early career, what regrets do you have about choices you made then that you wish you'd done differently in retrospect (i.e., what errors of commission did you make)?
3. Knowing me as you do, what biases or errors in my potential judgments about early career decision making should I be guarding against?

## REFERENCES

Ellis A, Harper RA: A Guide to Rational Living, 3rd Edition. North Hollywood, CA, Wilshire Books, 1975
Greenblatt M: Psychopolitics. New York, Grune and Stratton, 1978
Linn LS, Yager J, Cope D, et al: Health status, job satisfaction, job stress, and life satisfaction among academic and clinical faculty. JAMA 254:2775–2782, 1985
Linn LS, Yager J, Cope D, et al: Health habits and coping behaviors among practicing physicians. West J Med 144:484–489, 1986

## ADDITIONAL RESOURCES

**Sources for personal growth**
Covey SR, Merrill AR, Merrill RR: First Things First: To Live, to Love, to Learn, to Leave a Legacy. New York, Simon and Schuster, 1994
Csikszentmihalyi M: Finding Flow: The Psychology of Engagement With Everyday Life. New York, Basic Books, 1997

Nadler G, Hibino S: Breakthrough Thinking, 2nd Edition. Rocklin, CA, Prima Publishing, 1998

Sher B: I Could Do Anything If I Only Knew What It Was: How to Discover What You Really Want and How to Get It. New York, Dell Publishing, 1994

Sher B, Gottlieb A: Wishcraft: How to Get What You Really Want. New York, Ballantine Books, 2003

**Sources for early career building**

American Psychiatric Association resources for early career psychiatrists: http://www.psych.org/ecp/index.cfm

American Medical Association resources for early career physicians (for members): http://www.ama-assn.org/ama/pub/category/1963.html

American College of Medical Practice Executives: http://www.mgma.com/acmpe/index.cfm

*In addition, Google offers entry to an entire world of subspecialty organizations offering early career and mentorship programs, online M.B.A., medical executive courses, and other useful online instruction.*

*Through "A Short Postgraduate Reading Course in Administration and Management," the American Medical Association offers many books for the novice, including:*

Daigrepont JP, Mink L: Starting a Medical Practice, 2nd Edition. Chicago, IL, American Medical Association, 2003

Rainer C: Practice Management: A Practical Guide to Starting and Running a Medical Office. Lima, OH, Wyndham Hall Press, 2004

Reeves CS: Managing the Medical Practice, 2nd Edition. Chicago, IL, American Medical Association, 2002

**General introductions to administration**

Allen K, Economy P: The Complete MBA for Dummies. New York, Hungry Minds, 2000

Drucker PF: The Essential Drucker: The Best of Sixty Years of Peter Drucker's Essential Writings on Management. New York, Harper Business, 2003

Silbiger SA: The Ten-Day MBA: A Step-by-Step Guide to Mastering the Skills Taught in America's Top Business Schools. New York, William Morrow, 1999

**Sources for dealing with difficult supervisors, colleagues, and subordinates**

Berne E: Games People Play: The Psychology of Human Relationships. New York, Grove Press, 1964

Bernstein AJ, Rozen SC: Dinosaur Brains: Dealing With All Those Impossible People at Work. New York, Ballantine Books, 1989

Bernstein AJ, Rozen SC: Neanderthals at Work: How People and Politics Can Drive You Crazy and What You Can Do About Them. New York, Ballantine Books, 1992

Bramson RM: Coping With Difficult People: In Business and in Life. New York, Ballantine Books, 1981

Brinkman R, Kirshner R: Dealing With People You Can't Stand. New York, McGraw-Hill, 1994

Jacques E: Requisite Organization: A Total System for Effective Managerial Organization and Managerial Leadership for the 21st Century. Gloucester, MA, Cason Hall, 1988

Patterson K, Grenny J, McMillan R, et al: Crucial Conversations: Tools for Talking When Stakes Are High. New York, McGraw-Hill, 2002

Solomon M: Working With Difficult People. Upper Saddle River, NJ, Prentice-Hall, 2002

**An alternative perspective**

Bing S: What Would Machiavelli Do? New York, HarperCollins, 2002

**Sources for self-management**

*Time management*

MacKenzie RA, MacKenzie A: The Time Trap: The Classic Book on Time Management, 3rd Edition. New York, AMACOM , 1997

Morgenstern J: Time Management From the Inside Out: The Foolproof System for Taking Control of Your Schedule and Your Life. New York, Henry Holt, 2000

*Mood and affect management*

Ellis A, Harper R: A Guide to Rational Living, 3rd Edition. Los Angeles, CA, Wilshire, 1975

Ellis A: How to Stubbornly Refuse to Make Yourself Miserable About Anything—Yes, Anything. New York, Citadel, 1988

*Balancing career and work*

Keyes R: Timelock: How Life Got So Hectic and What You Can Do About It. New York, Random House, 1994

Ornstein R, Sobel DS: Healthy Pleasures. New York, Perseus, 1988

# Index

*Page numbers printed in **boldface** type refer to tables, figures, or appendices.*